Springer-Verlag Italia Srl.

A. Fortuna
L. Ferrante
P. Lunardi

Essential Illustrated Neurosurgery

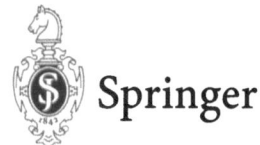

Springer

ALDO FORTUNA M.D.
Chairman of Neurosurgery
Director of the Neurosurgery Specialization School
Department of Neurosciences
University of Rome La Sapienza

LUIGI FERRANTE M.D.
Professor of Neurosurgery
Lecturer of Operative Technique
Neurosurgery Specialization School
Department of Neurosciences
University of Rome La Sapienza

PIERPAOLO LUNARDI
Professor of Neurosurgery
Lecturer of Operative Technique
Neurosurgery Specialization School
University of Rome Tor Vergata

Title of original edition:
Neurochirurgia Essenziale Illustrata. © *1999 Verduci Editore, Roma*
Note to the reader:
This book is being published also in Chinese under the ISBN 7-81072-150-X/R·145

© Springer-Verlag Italia 2001
Originally published by Springer-Verlag Milan in 2001.
Softcover reprint of the hardcover 1st edition 2001
ISBN 978-88-470-2910-1   ISBN 978-88-470-2908-8 (eBook)
DOI 10.1007/978-88-470-2908-8
Library of Congress Cataloging-in-Publication Data: applied for

Cover design: Simona Colombo
Typesetting and layout: Photo Life, Vimodrone, Milan

SPIN: 10781789

Preface

This book was born out of thirty years of didactic and practical experience with the intention of giving the reader concise neurosurgical elements and an appropriate selected iconography. This text wants to represent a practical and essential guide for the medical student and a useful reference point for specialists interested in pursuing more detailed literature studies. General practitioners and specialists in related subjects can consult this text to formulate a diagnosis and elaborate a proper therapy.

November, 2000   *The Authors*

Contents

1. Cranial dysraphias

With the words "status dysraphicus" we mean all central nervous system malformations consequent to the lack of fusion of the neural groove edges along the posterior midline.

Arnold-Chiari malformation

Arnold-Chiari malformation consists in the downward displacement of the primitive rhomboencephalon and herniation through the foramen magnum of the cerebellum and brainstem, which localize in the spinal canal with consequent compression. Chiari distinguished three types of malformations: type I is a simple downward dislocation of the cerebellar tonsils; type II also presents brainstem involvement; type III consists of an encephalocele which contains the subtentorial structures.

All the theories proposed to explain this lesion can be summarized as follows: 1) a progressive traction of the craniospinal junction due to a downward attachment of the medullary cord; 2) in case of hydrocephalus associated with a small posterior cranial fossa, the pressure from the top can cause the migration of the cerebellar tonsils to the occipital foramen; 3) a cerebellar and brainstem primary malformation; or 4) a basicranium malformation.

Williams, instead, underlined the importance of the pressure gradient between the intracranial and spinal compartments: during Valsalva's maneuver, an obstruction of the epidural veins should occur so as to cause subarachnoid space compression. In this way, the cerebrospinal fluid should be pushed toward the intracranial compartment. When the spinal venous pressure returns to normal levels, an opposite flow toward the spinal compartment should occur. If this balancing process fails because of adherences at the level of the occipital foramen, a pressure gradient forms between the two compartments, so that the cerebrospinal fluid will try to find its way through the obex causing a downward compression of the cerebellar tissue (Fig. 1.1a).

In the majority of newborns affected by a type II malformation, an obstructive hydrocephalus is present. They can present a laryngeal stridor, vocal cord paralysis, sudden asphyxia or dysphagy. These symptoms are due to the compressive action of the malformation on the brainstem at the level of the occipital foramen or the vertebral canal. The rapid decompression of the occipital foramen and of the first two cervical vertebrae is followed by their rapid regression.

The type I malformation is rarely symptomatic in newborns, manifesting itself during adolescence or adulthood. The symptomatology in older children and in adults is similar, the most frequent symptoms being ataxia, occipital pain, pain along the occipital nerve, hyposthenia of the four limbs, and positional primary nystagmus.

The radiological diagnosis is obtained with cerebral CT and NMR, which show herniation of the cerebellar tonsils through the foramen magnum with cervical compression (Fig. 1.1b) as far as the C2-C3 segments. In some cases the brainstem is also displaced downward, forcing the bulb and the fourth ventricle to localize at the level of the cervical space. CT and NMR can further reveal associated malformations: posterior cranial fossa smaller than normal, congenital stenosis of the Sylvian aqueduct, hydrocephalus, syringomyelia, basicranial malformations (platybasia, basilar impression), or microgyria.

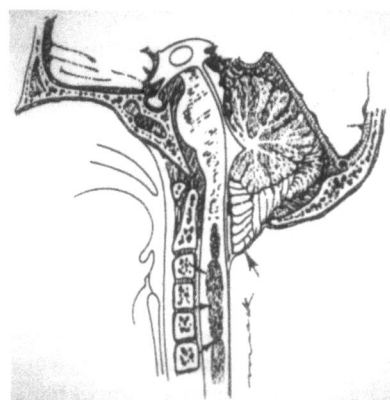
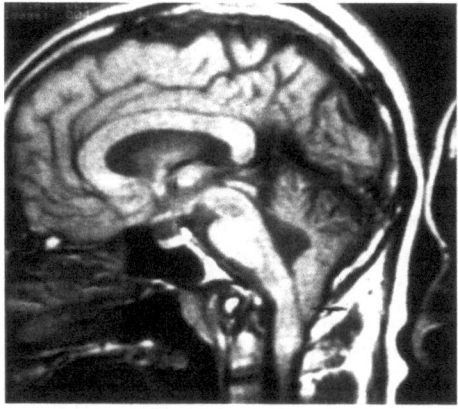

a   b

Fig. 1.1a,b. Arnold-Chiari malformation. **a** Exemplifying scheme. **b** NMR, T1 sagittal view. Cerebellar tonsils have herniated through the occipital foramen and compress the bulb and spinal cord

The surgical operation consists of the osseous decompression of the foramen magnum and first cervical vertebrae, and of the treatment of the hydrocephalus by a shunt application, i.e. fourth ventricle shunt and duraplasty. It also consists of the opening of the fourth ventricle foramina and closure of the communication between the obex and the central spinal canal. An association between this type of malformation and scoliosis, with or without a syringomyelic cavity, is well known. Carmel had already noticed that surgical treatment of the hydromyelocele can lead to an improvement in the neurological deficit and a decrease in severity of the scoliosis.

Dandy-Walker malformation

Dandy-Walker (DW) is a congenital malformation of the posterior cranial fossa, a cerebellar dysraphia due to the lack of fusion of the vermis during embryogenesis with imperforation of Magendi and Luschka's foramina and tetraventricular hydrocephalus. The clinical picture is characterized by signs and symptoms of intracranial hypertension. Newborns are often asymptomatic, presenting the first symptoms three months after birth. The symptoms can be: irritability, vomit, lethargy, encephalomegaly, tension of the fontanels, diastasis of the sutures, ataxia and nystagmus. In rare cases a meningocele (herniation of the meninges), an encephalocele (herniation of the meninges and cerebral tissue) or an encephalocystomeningocele (herniation of the encephalon, meninges and ventricles) can be observed. Other extracerebral anomalies such as cardiac defects, extremity malformations, visceral anomalies and facial angiomas are frequently present.

The differential diagnosis must be effected with an arachnoid cyst, a megacistern magna, or a cerebellar cystic tumor. Even if the ultrasonography has become highly dependable and can show the DW cyst in a fetus in utero, CT and NMR give more information about the presence of other anomalies such as corpus callosum agenesis (30% of cases) or poroencephalia. The radiological characteristics of a DW malformation are a partial or complete absence of the vermis cerebelli, a cystic dilation of the fourth ventricle, an enlarged posterior cranial fossa with an high insertion of the tentorium, and a hypoplasia of one or both of the cerebellar hemispheres (Fig 1.2a,b). The study of liquoral dynamics is essential to plan the type of surgical procedure. The first objective of the surgical operation is the treatment of the hydrocephalus.

Although the application of a ventriculoperitoneal shunt may seem a simple solution, it is not always advantageous. In fact, in case of obstruction

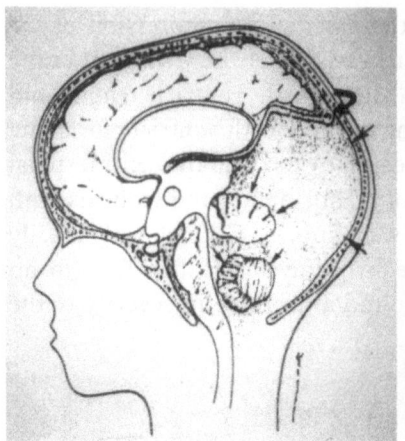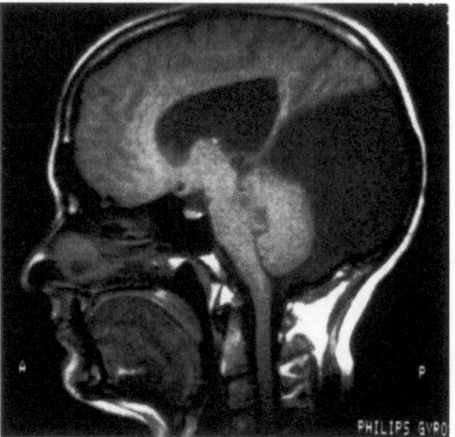

a   b

Fig.1.2a,b. Dandy-Walker malformation. Exemplifying cartoon (**a**) and MR, T1-weighted image, sagittal view (**b**). Diffuse cerebrospinal fluid accumulation in the posterior cranial fossa in direct continuity with the fourth ventricle and upward displacement of the tentorium. Cerebellar hypoplasia

of the aqueduct, there can be an upward herniation of the posterior cranial fossa contents. A cystoperitoneal shunt could, however, decrease the pressure in the posterior cranial fossa, causing a downward transtentorial hernia. A double cystoventriculoperitoneal shunt is also useful in some patients but ineffective in others, because the two shunts might not work in the same way. Better results are achieved with a solution that implies the connection of the two proximal tubings (cyst and ventricle) to a single reservoir. The main causes of death in patients affected by a DW malformation are shunt infections and cardiorespiratory arrest, due to brainstem malformation. The long-term results after surgical treatment reveal that some patients have normal intelligence, but others show signs of subnormal intelligence, especially if other anomalies, such as corpus callosum agenesis, are present.

Encephalocele

Encephalocele is the protrusion of the cranial contents (meninges, nervous tissue, ventricular cavities) through an osseous defect (bifid skull). The cranial dysraphism is less frequent than the spinal one and its incidence is about 1 in 3000-10 000 births. 0 occipital and frontobasal regions are more frequently affected.

In the *occipital encephalocele*, the cranial defect is on the midline, most often under the external occipital protuberance. The basis of the dural sac is strictly connected with the sagittal sinus, the torcularis sinus and the lateral sinuses. The sac is covered with normal skin (or with angiomatous-like skin) and its contents can be formed either by simple meninges or by a varying quantity of cerebral tissue. This tissue can be constituted by the hypoplasic cerebellar hemispheres with consequent brainstem strain and cranial nerve stretching, or by the occipital lobe. In this case, the surgeon must consider that the brain tissue can be histologically normal and still functional. This malformation can present anomalies of the optic nerves, the chiasm, the corpi quadrigemini and the brainstem; this can explain the variety of the neurological deficits observed in surviving patients .

The occipital encephalocele is a median, sessile or pedunculated swelling (Fig. 1.3a). Its dimensions are not informative of the sac contents;

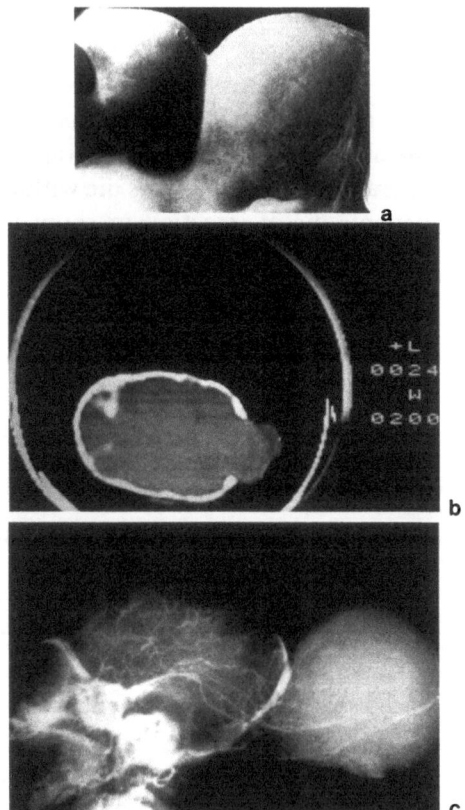

Fig. 1.3a-c. Occipital meningo-encephalocele (a). CT, axial view (b) and cerebral angiography (c). Extensive connection of the cranial theca with herniated cerebral tissue, vascularized by middle and posterior cerebral artery branches

only a sessile sac can affect the first occipital arch and it contains nervous tissue more frequently than a pedunculated sac. A microcephalic skull with a big sessile sac has a poor prognosis since most of the nervous tissue is contained in the encephalocele sac.

CT and NMR can give precious information since they reveal both the nature of the sac contents and other associated anomalies (Fig. 1.3b). It is important to complete the tests with a study of the cerebral spinal fluid (CSF) dynamics and with angiography which reveals if there are important vessels inside the sac (Fig. 1.3c). To evaluate if the cerebral tissue inside the occipital encephalocele is functional, we can perform EEG or visual evoked potentials of the sac. Their absence can indicate either a visual cortex alteration or an optic pathway alteration. The surgical operation aims to remove the sac without damaging the healthy cerebral tissue and to impermeably close the dura mater. In case of a microcephalic child without neurological deficit, but with a sac containing cerebellar tissue and brainstem, it is convenient to forsake the surgical operation. In case of an encephalocele with a modest osseous defect and a pedunculated sac, the anatomy of the malformation is quite simple, while a sessile sac located in the occipitocervical region is easily in contact with great venous vessels. If the herniated cerebral tissue has a normal aspect, but it cannot be put back into the cranial cavity, it becomes necessary to widen the bony defect and close the skin back, without damaging the nervous tissue. Without a surgical operation, 90% of patients die within a few months, while 14% of operated patients die of infection or shunt failure. The surviving patients have a physical and mental development depending on the quantity of nervous tissue contained in the cyst and on the subsequent hydrocephalus, observed in 30% of cases.

Frontoethmoidal encephaloceles and encephaloceles of the basal regions are less common and are differently named according to the osseous defect or the cyst localization. Frontoethmoidal encephaloceles are classified into: nasofrontal type (the external sac is pedunculated and situated either on the glabella or on the nose root); naso-ethmoidal type (compared to the previous one, the sac is situated in a lower part and it is usually sessile); or naso-orbital type (the mass can be mono- or bilateral and can occupy the inferior and medial parts of the orbital cavity displacing the ocular globi upwards and externally). Usually, the nervous tissue contained in these sacs is not viable and these lesions must be distinguished from other masses such as nasal gliomas, hemangiomas and dermoid cysts.

Cranial base encephaloceles are distinguished into *frontosphenoidal* (they extend through a defect of the sphenoidal wing, through the optic foramen or through the orbital fissure) and *transethmoidal* or *sphenoeth-*

moidal forms. These lesions do not show any external signs. They cause respiratory difficulty and rhinoliquorrhea, and sometimes they can be confused with nasal polyps. The investigative radiological tests are the same as for the occipital encephaloceles.

Surgical operation is necessary to close the dural sac in an impermeable way, to reconstruct the osseous defect and to repair eventual craniofacial anomalies, which are frequent in the frontoethmoidal form. The intracranial approach is preferable to repair basal and frontoethmoidal encephaloceles, while extracranial repair is possible only for the purely frontal encephaloceles or for the nasofrontal type of the frontoethmoidal group.

Cranial dermic sinus

The cranial dermic sinus is a connection between the scalp and the intracranial cavity covered by epithelium. It can form in every location, from the nasion to the occipital foramen, but it is more frequently found at the level of the external occipital protuberance. It can terminate in the subcutaneous tissue or it can penetrate, through a cranial defect, up to the epidural or intradural space. In 89% of cases, it is associated with a dysembryogenetic tumor, such as a dermoid cyst or a teratoma, which can be intra- or extradural. At the level of the nasion, the dermic sinus can be associated with a tumor situated in the ethmoid sinuses. If it extends through the cribiform lamina, the tumor can develop close by the diencephalic region.

In 84% of cases, this malformation occurs within 5 years of age and appears like a small cutaneous orifice without hairs and with angiomatous color. Patients can be asymptomatic or they can develop meningitis. In some cases an abscess can be present in the tumoral mass itself.

Patients affected by dermic sinus must undergo CT and NMR. These tests are able to show the intracranial masses, their anatomical relationships and a possible hydrocephalus. In case of meningitis, a cerebrospinal fluid culture is necessary to identify the pathological agent. The surgical operation aims at the complete removal of the dermic sinus and the dysembryogenetic tumor, if present. Removal of only the extracranial portion of the sinus is not sufficient to prevent the successive onset of meningitis or a tumor.

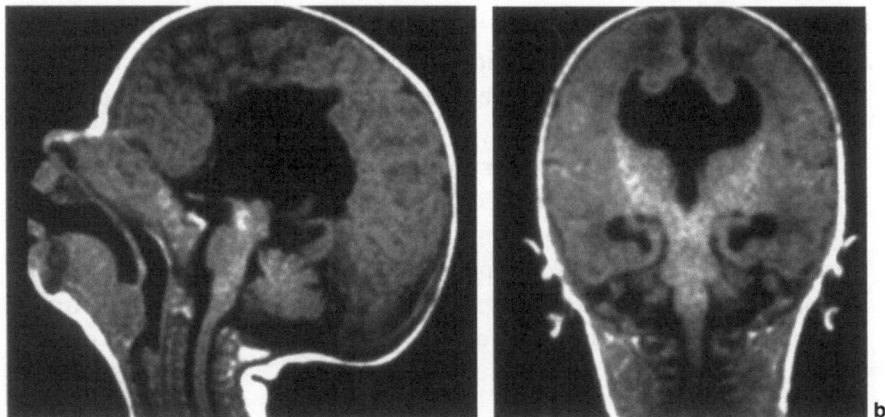

a

b

Fig.1.4a,b. Agenesis of the corpus callosum. NMR, T1-weighted images, sagittal (**a**) and coronal (**b**) views

Corpus callosum agenesis

This is the most frequent of the anterior dysraphias and it is associated with some other malformations. The symptomatology is variable and mainly due to the associated malformations. The most frequent symptoms are psychomotor retardation and generalized or partial convulsions. The diagnosis is based on CT and NMR images showing partial or complete absence of the corpus callosum (Fig. 1.4a,b).

2. Brain tumors

Epidemiology

The incidence of primary cerebral tumors varies in relation to the geographical areas considered. The countries more developed, from a socio-economic point of view, show a higher incidence compared to underdeveloped countries: the annual incidence of primary brain tumors in Sweden is about 10:100 000, while in China and India it is less than 2:100 000. The high incidence in some countries cannot be easily explained by differences in the healthcare or social systems. In fact, a highly developed country like Japan presents about a third of the cases observed in USA, suggesting the presence of a genetic predisposition in the American population.

Men are more affected than women, although meningiomas are more frequent in the latter group. The annual incidence of gliomas is 6-7 per 100 000 inhabitants, while the incidence of meningiomas is 3-4:100 000.

Recent studies have revealed an increase of primary cerebral tumors in elderly people. This can be explained by the recent and more frequent employment of noninvasive neuroradiological techniques and by an increase in the life span. Moreover, cerebral neoplasias constitute the most common type of neoplasia during pediatric age. If we consider children (under 15 years of age at the time of diagnosis) affected by primary cerebral tumors, we notice that 23% is affected by medulloblastoma, 25% by astrocytoma of low degree, 12% by cerebellar astrocytoma, 11% by cerebellar astrocytoma of high grade, and 9% by a brainstem glioma.

Symptoms and signs

The cerebral tumor symptomatology can be general, i.e. mainly due to an intracranial hypertension syndrome, or focal and specific due to irritative, compressive or destructive effects caused by the tumor on the cerebral parenchyma, or general and focal at the same time.

Intracranial hypertension

Headache

Headache is the initial symptom in one-third of patients affected by cerebral tumor: the pain, in the initial phase, is moderate, intermittent, and more accentuated in the early morning (the intracranial pressure is more elevated in the morning than during other parts of the day due to the overnight supine position and nocturnal hypercapnia even in healthy conditions), during physical efforts and during rapid movements of the head. It is caused by the stretching of the sensory nerve fibers of the dura mater and of the blood vessels.

During the initial period, the distribution and the clinical characteristics of the headache may indicate the location of the tumor. Headache limited to the occipital region with desultory episodes of frontal irradiation is a sign of a posterior cranial fossa tumor. Unilateral headache is characteristic of a supratentorial tumor. Headache which strikes with brief paroxystic fits of strong intensity is characteristic of isolated tumors in the ventricles, especially in the third one.

Vomit

Vomit is a symptom connected to intracranial hypertension, while less frequently it is caused by a direct involvement of the vagal nucleus or of the area postrema on the floor of the bulbar triangle of the fourth ventricle in injuries of the posterior cranial fossa. It is not preceded by nausea or related to meals, and it may be "projectile". It is not followed by that sense of exhaustion frequent in the vomit of gastric origin, and it is more frequent in morning on an empty stomach.

It is called "easy vomiting" and may be provoked by sudden changes of head position. In children, vomit may appear together with vague abdominal pains and be mistaken for vomit caused by acetonemia or by appendicitis.

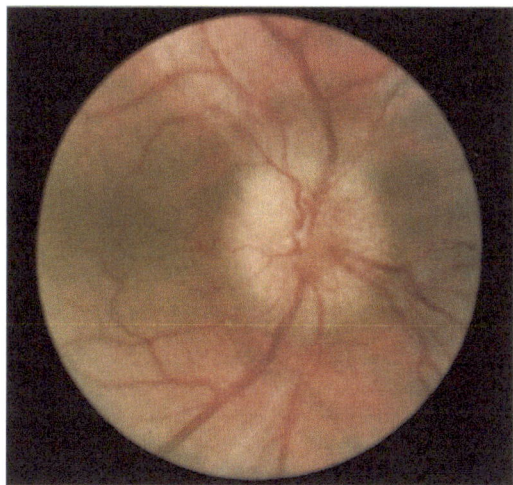

Fig. 2.1. Papilledema

Papillary stasis

It is due to a laborious venous circulation in the eye consequent to intracranial hypertension. It is characterized by swelling and protrusion of the optic papilla with blurry or absent margins and it is often bilateral with retinal hemorrhages (Fig. 2.1).

Vision remains normal for a long time. Visual impairment is minimal but momentary blackouts can occur for a few seconds. On the other hand, the narrowing of the visual fields and the increase in dimension of the blind spot are more precocious signs. In tumors of the anterior cranial fossa, peripapillary retinal edema with blurry margins and limited swelling

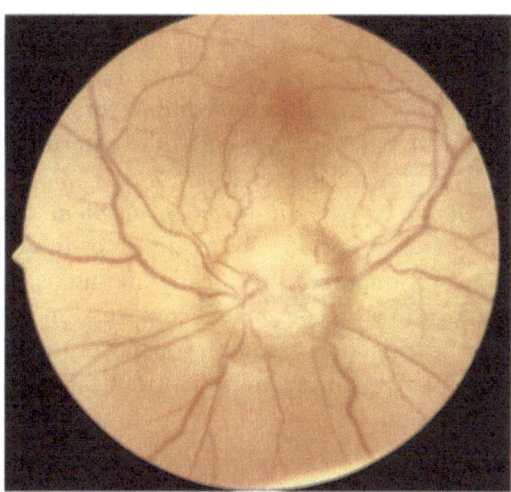

Fig. 2.2. Secondary optic atrophy

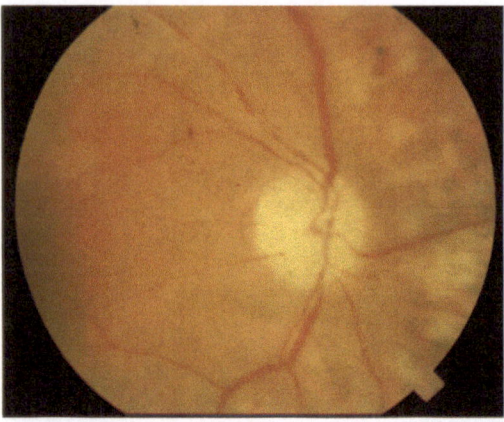

Fig. 2.3. Primary optic atrophy

is more frequent. The papillary stasis may be unilateral, and is sometimes associated with contralateral optic atrophy (Forster-Kennedy's syndrome) due to the direct compression of the optic nerve, as also happens in olfactory meningioma.

With further evolution of the disease, vision disappears, the hemorrhages are reabsorbed and the optic papillae become pale with blurry margins (secondary optic atrophy) (Fig. 2.2). In primitive optic atrophy (Fig. 2.3), optic papillae are pale, even if the margins are sharp.

Wedge or herniation

It represents a serious complication of intracranial hypertension in relation to the compression of important nervous structures. The most common and serious herniations are temporal and cerebellar. The transfalcial herniation, in which the cingulate gyrus is pushed under the falx, is characteristic of large, invasive frontal lesions. It does not show any characteristic clinical manifestation and it worsens the symptoms of the frontal syndrome due to compression of the anterior cerebral arteries and of the contralateral hemisphere.

Tentorial herniation or engagement may occur for all supratentorial tumors and, specifically, for those of the temporal lobe: the hippocampal convolution, more specifically the uncus, protrudes into the hiatus of the tentorium with consequent compression of the brainstem and homolateral third cranial nerve, complete palsy of the third cranial nerve, contralateral hemiparesis, and alteration of the state of consciousness. If the herniation is not reduced, a state of decerebration may appear, together with arterial hypertension and signs of bulbar stress, bradycardia, tachypnea or bradypnea, hyperthermia and death due to cardiorespiratory arrest.

In cases of slow herniation-compression, during the initial phase, the brainstem can be pushed against the opposite free edge of the tentorium with consequent contralateral pyramidal tract compression and appearance of a motor syndrome leading to the wrong localization of the lesion.

Cerebellar herniation or cerebellar tonsil engagement is a common feature of posterior cranial fossa tumors, but it may also be observed in supratentorial tumors. It is characterized by the herniation of the cerebellar tonsils in the occipital foramen. This herniation is responsible for bulb compression and for impairment of the cerebrospinal fluid circulation with subsequent increase of the intracranial pressure.

During the initial phase, the syndrome is characterized by intense occipitonuchal pain, neck stiffness, hypertonia of the nuchal muscles with the head forced in hyperextension, and is followed by opisthotonos crises with stiffening of the four limbs in extension (decerebration crisis), vomit, hiccup, arterial hypertension, bradycardia, bradypnea and death due to cardiorespiratory arrest.

Focal symptoms and signs

Epilepsy

Epilepsy is defined as a paroxystical hypersynchronism of a group of neurons adjacent to an injury, called focus, of variable dimensions, that typically leads to loss of consciousness. When the epileptic crises occur suddenly during adult or mature age, they are most likely the symptom of a cerebral tumor (unless other causes can be found).

Antiepileptic therapy, if the presence of a tumor is not suspected (the electroencephalogram can be normal), may be effective but it eliminates the possibility of an early diagnosis.

Epilepsy due to an invasive lesion is the least frequent and together with epilepsy due to scars (divided by Penfield into corticomeningeal scars and localized cortical atrophies) derived from traumas or infections, constitutes about 25% of cases. The essential epilepsies, whose etiology is unknown, are responsible for the remaining 75% of cases.

Generalized epileptic crises
Tonicoclonic crises from the start. Manifest as patients cry and fall to the ground with loss of consciousness. This is followed by the tonic phase with a stiffening in extension, with or without tremors, and finally by the clonic phase with bilateral and synchronous clonic jerks, drooling, and urine loss.

The recovery phase lasts many minutes and the appearance of automatic reflexes precedes the return to consciousness.

It is possible that this crisis of "grand mal epilepsy" arises from the centrencephalon, but it may be connected to a cortical focus with subsequent action on the centrencephalon.

Tonicoclonic crises that successively become genaralized represent the consequence of an initial symptom called "aura", which represents the real beginning of the crisis. The nature of the aura allows one to establish the exact location of the focus more precisely than by EEG (the word aura was coined by Galeno because the subject often felt a sort of breath a few seconds before the attack). An accurate anamnestic evaluation of the aura is important because it allows the diagnosis of symptomatic epilepsy: a visual hallucination indicates the occipital region as the origin of the crisis, while total or partial paresthesias of a limb or of part of it indicate the postrolandic sensory areas.

Petit mal epilepsy are characterized by brief loss of consciousness, a glassy stare without falling to the ground. Often they are accompanied by palpebral clonus or by synchronized upward deviation of the gaze, the head and the eyes. Exceptional muscular contractions in the face and lower limbs or automatic activities are present. This is particularly frequent during childhood.

Myoclonic minor epilepsy is similar to the precedent with abrupt myoclonias of the upper limbs and sometimes of the lower limbs.

Akinetic minor epilepsy causes an abrupt block of postural tone with flaccid fall to the ground.

Partial seizures

They are characterized by symptoms relative to limited sensory and motor structures, without loss of consciousness. We can distinguish simple partial crises and complex partial crises.

Simple partial crises

Somatomotor or jacksonian crises are rhythmic clonus of a muscular group sometimes limited to a finger or to some facial muscles, and they often spread into the adjacent motor areas according to the cortical somatotopy (jacksonian march). After a crisis, a transient motor deficit remains but there is no loss of consciousness and the subject is aware of the attack. They indicate the localization of the lesion. In adult patients, the most frequent causes are cerebral tumors, head traumas and cerebral MAV.

Adversative tonic crises are characterized by a synchronized tonic deviation of the head and eyes toward the opposite side of the lesion. In some cases, the abduction and elevation of the upper limb semiflexed to the elbow with a closed fist is observed.

Crises with vocalization or crises of the supplemental motor area are characterized by elevation of the contralateral upper limb with repetitive vocalization.

Somatosensory crises are similar to dysesthesias (sensation of pricking, tingling, numbness). They may be localized to one thumb, one hand, one limb, one foot, a lower limb, part of the body, or one half of the face. They may spread to adjacent areas according to the cortical somatotopy. They indicate the localization of the lesion. The causes are similar to those of the somatomotor crises.

Visual crises are characterized by elementary visual sensations, like phosphenes, scotoma, variations of an object's dimension (micropsiae, macropsiae), deformation of the objects (metamorphopsiae). They are genuine aurae, and they may remain as such or give rise to a generalized crisis. The lesion is localized in the occipital area and it is accompanied by deficits of the visual field (partial or complete homonymous lateral hemianopsia).

Auditory crises cause elementary auditory sensations (whistles, bell and sounds), variations in the tone and volume of sounds. The simple forms are in relation to lesions of the transverse temporal convolution (Henschl's gyrus), while complex ones are part of psychomotor epilepsy.

Olfactory crises cause unpleasant olfactory sensations (burnt meat, rotten eggs) and represent aurae of more complex crises. They may cause olfactory illusions like decreased or increased perception of the perceived odors. The injury is localized in the temporal lobe, uncinate gyrus.

Olfactory-gustatory crises may be associated with the olfactory sensations previously described, inducing acidic, bitter or salty sensations. The lesion is localized in the anterior part of the temporal lobe, more specifically in the uncus, amygdala and hippocampus if the crises are olfactory or in the insula if the crises are gustatory.

Visceral crises. Oral crises (sucking, mastication, swallowing), epigastric crises (nausea, sternoepigastric sensations up to the throat), intestinal crises (colics, eructations, borborygmi) are in relation to the cortical somatosensory representation of the abdominal organs as shown by Penfield, during neurosurgical operations in which he stimulated Reil's insula. In general, they can be considered aurae of temporal epilepsy.

Hallucinatory crises often are multisensorial hallucinations that can be reproduced by stimulation of the temporal cortex in those areas involved in the consolidation and retrieval of memories. They are "deja vu"-like hallucinations, as we observe in temporal tumors.

Ictal automatisms may be simple or complex gestures (touching parts of the body, stripping, repeating work activities) or deambulatory automatisms (walking in and out of a room, covering large distances, the so-called epileptic escapes). They are characterized by a decrease in the state of consciousness and by no memory of the event, due to the interference of the temporal lobe imputs on the memory mechanisms. Penfield has experimentally reproduced them by stimulating the temporal lobe (amygdala, circuminsular temporal cortex, anterior hippocampus).

Vertiginous crises. The responsible lesion seems to be located in the temporal lobe, where a central representation of the labyrinthus seems to exist.

Complex partial crises

The classical denomination is epileptic equivalents or psychomotorial epilepsy, now called temporal epilepsy, since the temporal area is the most frequent location of the lesion. They can appear like minor psychomotorial crises, anticipated by emotional, sensorial, visceral or hallucinatory manifestations, brief loss of consciousness, sometimes oral automatisms, and complex gesture automatisms. In some cases they can appear like major psychomotor crises which begin, as the above, with multivarious aurae, often followed by crises of grand mal epilepsy.

Language disorders

Broca's aphasia is characterized by disorders of the spoken language which is badly articulated, slow, interrupted, and laborious. The localization of the lesion is on the foot of the left third frontal convolution or supplemental motor area, on the medial surface of the hemisphere. The aphasia can be the initial symptom of a frontal tumor, but it can also be associated with psychic or motor disorders.

Wernicke's aphasia is characterized by disorders in the comprehension of spoken and written language. It is accompanied by logorrhea, rich in paraphasies and unintelligible neologisms. The lesion is localized in the posterior part of the left first temporal convolution and in the inferior parietal lobule, namely in the supramarginal and angular gyrus.

Aphasic disorders due to left hemisphere tumors have a slow progression, similar to the circumscribed cerebral hemorrhages caused by head trauma, angioma and transient ischemic disorders.

Optic pathway disorders

Primary optic atrophy appears with a varying but permanent level of visual deficit. The optic disk has a pale appearance at ophthalmoscopic examination but there are well defined margins. The visual field examination can show a central scotoma.

The first possibility to take into consideration is an optic nerve compression. The pathological conditions which could cause it are numerous: optic nerve tumors, optic canal fractures, intraorbital hematomas, intraorbital tumors, craniofacial malformations (craniostenosis, Crouzon's disease), meningiomas of the lesser wing of the sphenoid bone, hypophysial tumors, parasellar tumors or aneurysms of the anterior communicating and internal carotid arteries. The optic nerve can be also

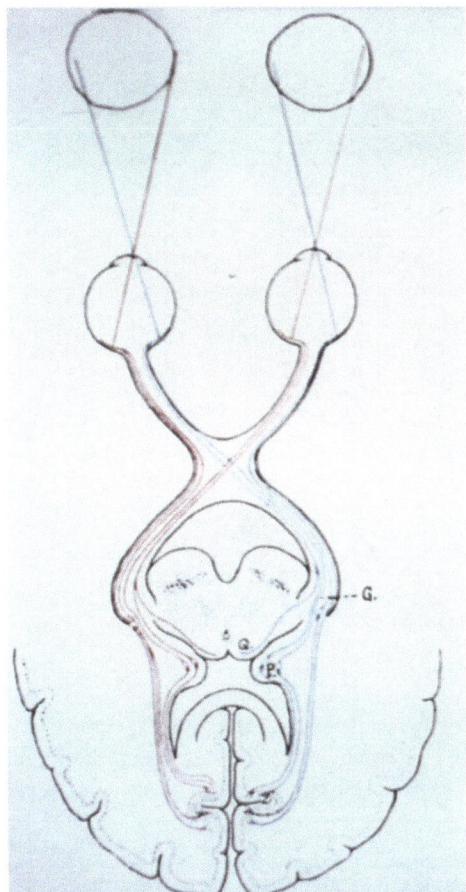

Fig. 2.4. The optic pathway

compressed by anterior cranial fossa tumors which, if causing intracranial hypertension, can be associated with contralateral papilledema (Forster-Kennedy's syndrome). The optic atrophy can be associated with chiasmatic lesions.

Chiasmatic lesions (Figs. 2.4; 2.5) The compression of the median part of the chiasm causes bitemporal hemianopsia (Fig. 2.6), namely visual loss in both temporal halves of the visual field. Because of the arrangement of the optic fibers in the chiasm, if the initial compression occurs from the top (for example in the saddle tubercle meningiomas), the visual loss in both temporal fields only affects the inferior half of each temporal field (inferior quadrantic temporal hemianopsia). On the contrary, when the compression occurs from below (for example in hypophyseal adenomas), a superior quadrantic temporal hemianopsia is observed.

Binasal hemianopsia consists of loss in both nasal halves. It is a rare condition, due to the bilateral lateromedial compression of the chiasm.

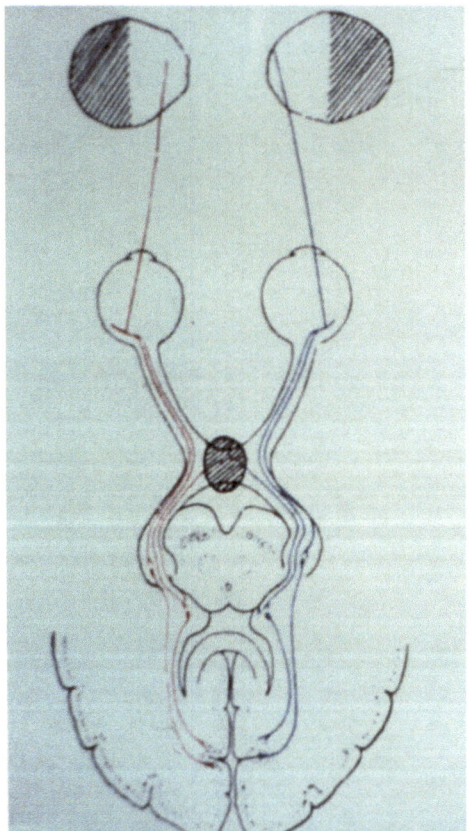

Fig. 2.5. Chiasmatic lesion: bitemporal hemianopsia

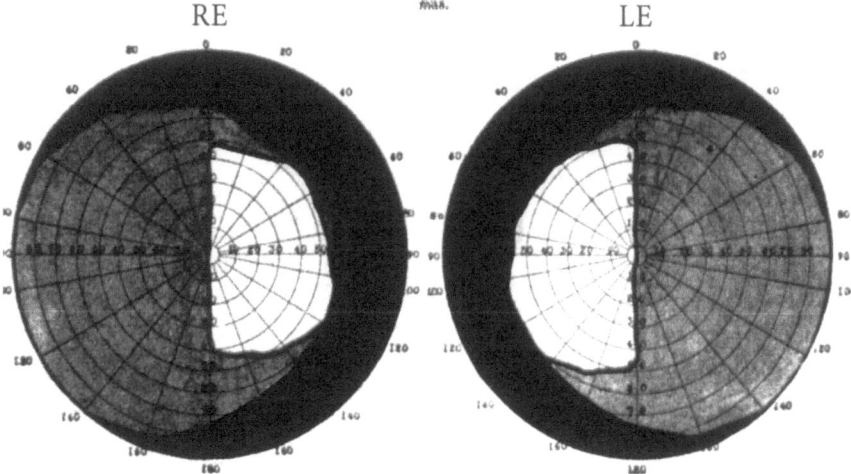

Fig. 2.6. Visual field: bitemporal hemianopsia. RE: right eye; LE: left eye

Retrochiasmatic lesions (Fig. 2.7)

Homonymous lateral hemianopsia is contralateral to the lesion and is characterized by visual loss in the temporal half of a field and in the nasal half of the opposite field (Fig. 2.8).

The visual acuity of both eyes is not damaged, because half of the fibers originating from the macula of each eye are spared from damage. The lesion is almost always a tumor which can affect the optic band, and the parietal, temporal and occipital optic radiations.

Homonymous lateral quadrantanopia occurs when the lesion is localized. It only involves the optic tracts of the parietal or temporal radiations (inferior quadrantic homonymous lateral quadrantanopia or superior quadrantic homonymous lateral quadrantanopia) (Fig. 2.9).

Cortical blindness is caused by bilateral lesions of the optic radiations or of the occipital cortical area. Tumors are rarely the cause.

Apraxias

Apraxia is the inability to carry out purposeful movements in the absence of paralysis or other motor or sensory impairment, especially the inability to make proper use of an object. It is a sign of corpus callosum and parietal lobe damage.

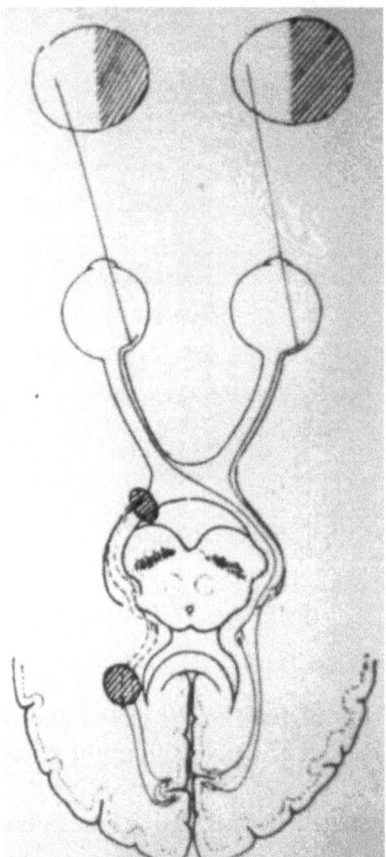

Fig. 2.7. Post-chiasmatic lesions: homonymous lateral hemianopsia

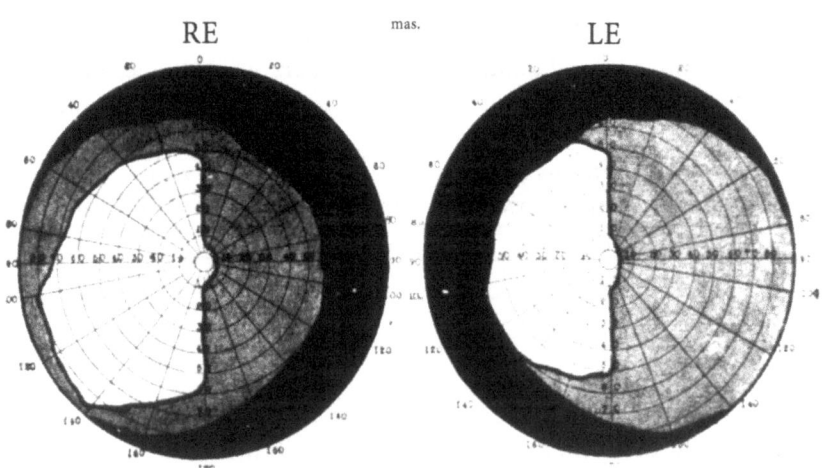

Fig. 2.8. Visual field: homonymous lateral hemianopsia. RE: right eye; LE: left eye

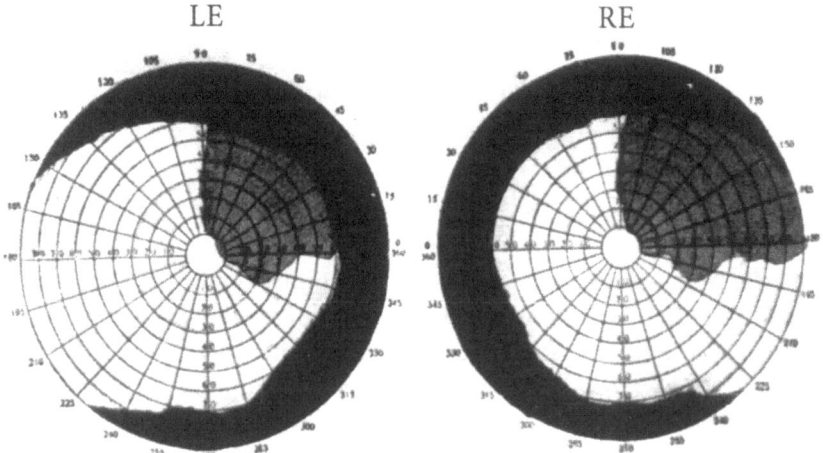

Fig. 2.9. Visual field: quadrantic homonymous lateral hemianopsia. LE: left eye; RE: right eye

Motor apraxia is characterized by the reduction of spontaneous movements with prevalence of the tone in the contralateral hemisoma. When the localization is prefrontal, grasping behavior can be observed.

Dynamic apraxia is an incapacity of performing planned movements (for example greeting with the hand, blowing a kiss). In dynamic apraxia, the lesion is frontal and the disorder is more intense on the left side.

Ideomotor apraxia in the incapacity or insufficient ability to perform simple or complex spontaneous movements, while they can be more or less imitated. The lesion is localized in the left parietal lobe.

Ideatory apraxia. The sequence of elementary gestures for the execution of the movements in complex actions is quite disturbed. For the most part it is associated with an ideomotor apraxia and the left parietal lobe is involved.

Constructive apraxia is a serious alteration in the perception of spatial relationships. Above all, it manifests itself during writing and sketching. It can be related to a lesion of the left parietal lobe.

Psychic disorders

The prefrontal tumors often begin with psychic symptoms, characterized by a progressive reduction of activity and attention, and short-term memory disorders, emotional indifference and disinterest. These symptoms are associated with a euphoric state and unmotivated excitement, as is characteristic of prefrontal lesions. Sometimes patients show an anomalous social behavior. Korsakoff's syndrome is characterized by anterograde amnesia and, in a minor way, by retrograde amnesia. The lesion involves the hippocampus-mammilo-thalamic circuit.

Cerebellar syndrome

Cerebellar dysmetria consists in the impossibility to correctly regulate the duration and the intensity of muscular action in relation to the object to be reached. Such disorder is revealed by the index-nose test.

Cerebellar ataxia is an irregularity and uncoordination of movements.

Adiadochocinesia consists of the incapability of performing rapid and alternate movements of pronation-supination with the hand. The disorder is revealed by beating the thigh alternatively with the palm and the back of the hand or alternatively turning the hand in horizontal position.

Hypotonia is a muscular tone modification or unequal tone distribution among agonist (hypotonic) and antagonist (hypertonic) muscles, therefore passive movements of the limbs are wider. The hypotonia leads to an exaggerated dangling of the hands and arms (ballottement sign).

Dyschronometry is a delay in the beginning or an excessive prolungation of a movement. It is easily evidenced by bringing both index fingers to the nose simultaneously.

Asynergic gait is expression of a spatial and temporal disharmony of the elementary muscular activities which cooperate to the movement execution. The patient brings ahead the lower limbs without measure, the foot falls down on the floor with force without bringing the trunk foreward. The phenomenon of retropulsion, which is corrected pushing the body ahead, is frequent.

Frontal lobe tumors

The tumors affecting this lobe lead to a polymorphic syndrome. Generally, the initial syndrome is psychic and is characterized by the difficulty to maintain attention and to assimilate new information. The patient becomes inactive, apathetic, abulic and, missing social inhibitions, can display inappropriate behavior. A supplemental motor area involvement in the frontal gyrus medial surface can provoke an epileptic seizure preceded by vocalizations and followed by increased muscular tone of the extremities.

The motor aphasia can be the result of damage to the Broca's area, situated on the foot of the second frontal convolution of the dominant hemi-sphere. In these cases, the association with agraphia is frequent. The involvement of the posterior part of frontal lobe, at the level of the pre-rolandic region, can cause a syndrome with motor deficit contralateral to the lesion, or an irritative motor syndrome in form of contralateral jack-sonian crises.

The beginning of the crises to the lower limbs or to the upper limbs indicates the site of the tumor in the median or inferior zone of the rolandic region, respectively.

Deep lesions affecting the corpus callosum and the gyrus cinguli induce urinary incontinence and more or less severe apathy. If the fronto-pontine fibers of the cortico-ponto-cerebellar system are affected, ataxia and dys-metria will be observed.

Parietal lobe tumors

In this region, like in the previous ones, gliomas are the most frequent tumors. Contralateral sensory hypoesthesia is the most frequent and char-acteristic sign. The different forms of sensitivity can be differentially affected; the proprioceptive sensitivity is the most involved. As a conse-quence, ataxia of the limb contralateral to the tumor becomes evident. This ataxia is different from cerebellar ataxia, because the symptom is increased by closing the eyes. There is a loss of the sense of position and of the spa-tial relationship of the extremities (asomatognosis). The patient may be incapable of recognizing the faces of relatives (prosopoagnosis), he has dif-ficulty in recognizing letters and numbers traced on the skin (graphoanes-thesia), and difficulty in recognizing objects to the touch (astereognosis).

In case of involvement of the dominant hemisphere, when the tumor is localized in the region of the angular gyrus, language disorders occur (sen-sorial aphasia or Wernicke's aphasia). Furthermore, Gerstmann's syn-drome, characterized by agraphia, acalculia, agnosia digitorum and confu-sion between right and left side, can occur.

Temporal lobe tumors

In temporal lobe tumors, the most frequent clinical manifestation is char-acterized by epileptic seizures called "temporal crisis" or "psychomotor crisis", due to the presence of simple or complex automatisms. The crises have different features according to the location of the tumor. For example, when the uncinate gyrus or uncus are affected, olfactory and disagreeable gustatory hallucinations, mastication movements, swallowing, and alterations of the state of consciousness with sensation of living strange and pleasant events (dreamy state) can occur.

These crises called "uncinate gyrus crises", are very informative for the localization of the tumor. In this region the symptomatology is rich and polymorphic: complex visual hallucinations with micropsia and macropsia, dreamy state, vision of complex scenes, detachment, déja vu, appearance of automatisms such as rubbing hands, unbuttoning, sucking, and mastication. In addition, auditory and vertiginous hallucinations can be present.

A lesion affecting the posterior part of the temporal lobe, in proximity to the calcarine cortex, can induce an epilepsy characterized by visual hallucinations and visual field alterations in form of contralateral superior and homonymous quadrantanopia. This evolves in complete homonymous lateral hemianopsia, with involvement of the central vision.

When the dominant hemisphere is damaged and the Wernicke's area is involved, language disorders appear in form of sensory aphasia: the patient loses comprehension of language, he can read and write phrases already written, but he does not understand the meaning of the words; the language is fluent, but incomprehensible due to errors and neologisms.

Psychic disorders are frequent mainly as character disorders, depressive disorders and psychic deterioration.

Occipital lobe tumors

The occipital lobe has modest dimensions and a tumor affecting this part of the brain often involves the neighboring temporal and parietal lobes, resulting in a complex symptomatology. An occipital lobe lesion can determine the onset of visual illusions or simple and complex hallucinations in the form of spots, bright rings, colored stripes, and alterations of dimension, form, color, and movement of objects. Multiple images of a single object can be perceived (palinopia). A visual field alteration is another symptom that is always present, in the form of quadrantanopia, followed by contralateral homonymous lateral hemianopsia with no damage to the macular vision. As a consequence, the central vision is preserved, making the hemianopsia less evident than that caused by the temporal tumors.

A frequent manifestation of an occipital lobe tumor is an epileptic crises in form of simple hallucinations in the contralateral visual field, sometimes evolving into a generalized crises.

Posterior cranial fossa tumors

In relation to their anatomical location, we can distinguish cerebellar tumors, fourth ventricle tumors, ponto-cerebellar angle tumors and brain-stem and clivus tumors.

Cerebellar tumors

The most frequent tumoral variety are astrocytomas, medulloblastomas, hemangioblastomas and metastases. These tumors are typical of pediatric and juvenile age, with the exclusion of the metastatic type.

The clinical picture shows signs of intracranial hypertension followed by secondary focal signs. Headache is the most frequent first symptom in 80%-90% of adults and in 70% of children. The headache is localized in the suboccipital region with nuchal and neck irradiations and sometimes with frontal region irradiation. In the initial phase of the disease the headache appears during the night (so painful that the patient wakes up), or during the early morning. It worsens with all activities that increase the intracranial pressure (physical efforts, cough, vomit). Vomit is a frequent symptom and in children it is present in 90% of the cases. It appears in the morning on an empty stomach, with or without nausea; it is explosive, induced by abrupt head movements, and abdominal pains can be present. Progressively, other intracranial hypertension signs appear: papillary stasis, diplopia, psychic disorders, and increasing of cranial diameter in children whose cranial sutures are not joined yet.

Focal symptoms

In tumors of the vermis, brainstem ataxia and walking disorders, evidenced by abrupt changes in direction, are frequent. The patient presents a widened support base, upper limbs away from the trunk, the head is kept still and slightly flexed forward.

In cerebellar hemisphere tumors, the symptomatology occurs with uncertain gait, a widened support base, the patient is inclined to skid and deflect toward to homolateral side of the tumor and he reacts shifting from the contralateral side (zig-zag gait or drunken gait); signs of motor disorganization are present, such as dysmetria, adiadochocinesia, asynergia and a notable hypotonia homolateral to the tumor.

In tumors compressing the dentate nuclei, intentional tremor is present.

Fourth ventricle tumors

See "Tumors of the cerebral ventricles".

Ponto-cerebellar angle tumors

The ponto-cerebellar angle is an arachnoid cistern of the posterior cranial fossa, limited by the petrous bone wall laterally, by the brainstem medially, by the cerebellum posterolaterally and by the tentorium rostrally.

Cranial nerves VI to XII are localized here, together with the superior petrous vein and the anterior-inferior and posterior-inferior cerebellar arteries.

The most frequent ponto-cerebellar angle tumors are: nerve VII neurinomas (80%-90%), meningiomas (5%-7%), dermoid and epidermoid tumors (3%-5%), nerve V neurinomas, metastases, arachnoid cysts, and aneurysms. The clinical characteristics of the ponto-cerebellar angle lesions are fairly specific.

The acoustic neurinoma has an insidious beginning of progressive unilateral hearing loss, usually within months or years, with tinkling, buzzing and water sounds, vertiginous sensation, equilibrium instability especially in scarcely illuminated places and appearence of nystagmus with slow jerks which beat on the tumor side.

During this phase, audiometric examination reveals a retrocochlear hypoacusis while the vestibular examination reveals homolateral vestibular hyporeflexia.

It is important to consider that in the absence of basic instrumental examinations, symptoms of hypoacusia with tinkling sounds and the absence or decrease of the homolateral corneal reflex (coexistent lesion of cranial nerve V) allow a clinical diagnosis. Evoked potentials show specific alterations (extension of the V wave). Cerebral CT and NMR, with contrast medium, evidence neurinomas of 2-3 mm in diameter.

Afterwards, with the growth of the neurinoma in the ponto-cerebellar angle, a variety of symptoms will start appearing: facial nerve paresis or spasm, cerebellar syndrome, dysphonia or dysphagia (deficit in the last cranial nerves).

Meningiomas are responsible for the same symptomatology but with some exceptions: the hearing loss is delayed, while the involvement of cranial nerve VII is more rapid, due to the fact that the meningioma often forms on the anterior margin of the internal acoustic meatus.

The radiological diagnosis is easily obtained with CT and cerebral NMR with contrast medium.

Brainstem tumors

They are infiltrating, not well-delimited tumors, mainly found during pediatric or juvenile age. The pons and the bulb are the most affected regions. The most frequent histological varieties are the gliomas, astrocytomas, glioblastomas, oligodendrogliomas, and ependymomas.

It is difficult to classify the symptomatology because of its complexity. The syndrome is characterized by various cranial nerve deficits in combination with ataxia and corticospinal tract deficits in the absence of intracranial hypertension. Cranial nerves V through XII are involved; cranial nerve IV is the first and the most frequently involved. Initially, corticospinal tract damage occurs with deep tendinous hyperreflexia and with clonus prevalently in the lower limbs, followed by spastic tetraparesis.

Clivus tumors

The clivus is localized in the median region of the basicranium and it delimits the anterior part of the posterior cranial fossa (PCF). The clivus is delimited posteriorly by the sphenoid bone and inferiorly by the basilar zone of the occipital bone. It contains important anatomical structures: brainstem, cranial nerves V to XII, and the vertebro-basilar vascular system.

The lesions involving the clivus are rare and they are classifed in extradural and intradural.

The extradural injuries can be benign (meningiomas, epidermoid cysts, cholesterinic granulomas), moderately malignant (chondroma and chondrosarcoma), or highly malignant (osteogenetic sarcoma, squamous cell tumors).

The most common benign intradural tumors are the meningiomas (representing 3%-10% of tumors in the PCF), the epidermoid cysts, the cranial nerve neurinomas, and the vertebro-basilar aneurysms.

In some cases, the anamnesis is characterized by headache and by involvement of cranial nerve V with pain, paresthesia, and hypoesthesia in the trigeminal territory; cranial nerve VI with diplopia; cranial nerve VII with peripheral paralysis or facial spasm; cranial nerve VIII with vertigo, hypoacusis, nystagmus; cranial nerves IX-X with dysphonia; and dysphagia; and cranial nerve XII with tongue paresis.

In other cases the clinical picture is characterized by pyramidal tract deficit like monoparesis, hemiplegia, spastic tetraparesis and by cerebellar signs like ataxia, asynergia, adiadochocinesia, dysmetria, and equilibrium disorders.

Generally, there is a progressive addition of various disorders culminating in an intracranial hypertension syndrome during the most advanced phase of the disease.

Tumors of the cerebral ventricles

Tumors of the lateral ventricles

These tumors are mostly benign, they grow slowly and reach big dimensions before becoming symptomatic. The most frequent varieties of tumors are the choroid plexi papilloma, ependymomas, subependymomas, meningiomas, teratomas, gliomas and metastases.

The symptomatology is characterized by an intracranial hypertension syndrome, due to an obstructive hydrocephalus or to a hypersecretive hydrocephalus, and by symptoms linked to the compression affecting the nearby regions (frontal, occipital, temporal, trigone horn). The initial symptomatology is quite vague, presenting headache, equilibrium disorders, and memory disorders. Afterwards, ataxia, visual deficit, hyperreflexia, apraxia and occasionally epilepsy can appear.

Third ventricle tumors

They are rare and present various symptoms and polymorphous signs in relation to their location and the anatomical structure affected. In relation to their location we distinguish: a) primary tumors of the third ventricle originating from structures forming the ventricular walls or from embryonic residues (colloid cysts, or astrocytomas, ependymomas, papillomas, craniopharyngiomas, teratomas, epidermoid and dermoid cysts, ependymal cysts, or parasitic cysts) and b) secondary tumors originating from the sellar or parasellar region (pituitary adenoma, craniopharyngioma, meningiomas, metastatic tumors).

The clinical picture is characterized by an intracranial hypertension syndrome, secondary to an obstructive hydrocephalus. The hypertensive crisis can be changed, increased or attenuated with changes in head position. Additionally, there can be memory disorders and signs of hypothalamic-pituitary axis damage (drowsiness, diabetes insipidus, appetite change, sleep-wake rhythm change, visual and campimetric deficit).

The tumors of the posterior part of the third ventricle are characterized by mydriasis, pupil rigidity and upward gaze restraint due to the quadrigeminus corpi and periaqueductal substance compression.

Fourth ventricle tumors

The fourth ventricle tumors can originate from the ventricular walls, the most frequent being the ependymomas and choroid plexi papillomas. If they originate from the nearby structures, like the vermis cerebelli, they are medulloblastoma or astrocytoma. These tumors, obstructing the fourth ventricle, induce hydrocephalus with intracranial hypertension syndrome presenting characteristic features: sudden crises of nuchal headache which spreads to the neck and shoulders and often caused by physical efforts and abrupt head movements. Patients hold their head in a forced position, slightly tilted forward.

This posture causes a characteristic gait, called "pageant gait". Afterwards, we can observe cerebellar or ponto-cerebellar angle symptoms (in case of lateral extension across the recess and Luska's and Magendi's foramina) and eventually brainstem deficit.

Pineal region tumors

These tumors originate from the pineal gland, or from other adjacent tissues, and they represent 1% of all intracranial tumors.

The tumor can originate from the parenchymal cells of the pineal gland (pinealoma, pineoblastoma), from the germinal cells (germinoma, teratoma, teratoid, embryonal carcinoma, choriocarcinoma) or from the glial cells (astrocytomas, glioblastomas, oligodendrogliomas). Epidermoid and dermoid cysts, meningiomas, metastases, arachnoid cyst and Galeno's ampulla aneurysms are quite rare.

The clinical picture is characterized by symptoms and signs of compression or invasion of the local structures. If the superior colliculi and the pretectal area are affected, we can observe upward gaze limitation (Parinaud's syndrome), pupil anomalies, paralysis of the convergence, retraction nystagmus, bilateral hyperacusis or hypoacusis. In case of sylvian aqueduct compression, an intracranial hypertension syndrome appears due to the obstructive hydrocephalus.

Compression and infiltration of the cerebellum cause dysmetria, ataxia, hypotonia and tremors. Cerebral CT and NMR with contrast medium allow the diagnosis of an expansive lesion of the pineal gland, while it is not always possible to determine the nature of the tumor.

Sellar and parasellar region tumors

The anatomical structures of these regions are formed by a bony component (sella turcica, tuberculum sellae, internal third of the wing of the sphenoid bone, superior part of the sphenoid fissure, superior third clivus, sphenoid sinus) and by glandular and neurovascular components (hypophysis, pituitary infundibulum, third ventricle anterior recess, optic nerves, optic chiasm, cavernous sini, neurovascular structures of the sphenoid fissure, cranial nerves II, IV and VI, trigeminal ophthalmic branch, and carotid arteries).

The most common pathologies are: hypophyseal adenomas, craniopharyngiomas, optic chiasm and hypothalamic gliomas, meningiomas, and aneurysms. The rarest pathologies are: empty sella syndrome (arachnoid cistern herniation in the sellar cavity due to hypoplasia or aplasia of the sellar diaphragm), arachnoid cyst, germinomas, nose-pharyngeal carcinomas, metastatic carcinomas, and chondroma.

In relation to the complexity of the anatomical structures forming this region, the clinical picture presents multiple and polymorphous symptoms and signs. The visual and campimetric deficits are useful for the localization of the lesion.

A syndrome showing visual and campimetric deficits is expression of lesions growing anteriorly: tuberculum and sphenoid planum meningiomas, non-secreting adenomas, and anterior communicating artery aneurysms.

The syndromes characterized by homonymous hemianopsia and bitemporal hemianopsia with scotoma are expression of optic tract or posterior chiasm compression (craniopharyngiomas, ectopic pinealoma, or superior third clivus tumors).

The unilateral visual deficit with optic atrophy is sign of a meningioma arising from the anterior clinoid process and the tuberculum or of a carotid-ophthalmic aneurysm. The presence of deficit of cranial nerves III-IV or VI, deficit of the trigeminal ophthalmic branch and exophthalmos can be expression of a meningioma of the third internal sphenoid wing or of the cavernous sinus.

Nonsecreting pituitary adenomas, during the period of intrasellar development, can be silent, while the pituitary adenomas of the secreting variety cause a purely endocrine symptomatology.

The prolactine-secreting adenomas (PRL) induce a syndrome of galactorrhea and amenorrhea.

The somatotropic adenoma (GH) leads to gigantism during the pediatric age or acromegaly in adults.

ACTH secreting adenoma is responsible for Cushing's disease. When the pituitary adenoma protrudes out of the sella turcica, we can observe signs of bitemporal hemianopsia and vision decrease due to chiasm and optic nerve compression.

With progressive growth of the tumor, a variety of symptoms develop: hypothalamic compression (diabetes insipidus, bulimia, hypersomnia, thermoregulation disorders, memory disorders), cavernous sinus compression (oculomotor nerves and trigeminal ophthalmic branch deficit) frontal and temporal lobe and brainstem compression, and intracranial hypertension syndrome due to the hydrocephalus caused by third ventricle compression.

The craniopharyngiomas developed from embryonic residue of Rathke's pouch (mainly of suprasellar origin) lead to hypophyseal insufficiency, hypothalamic compression, and optic-posterior compression with vision and visual field alterations.

Anatomopathological classification

Benign cerebral tumors (Tab. 2.1)

Leptomeningeal tumors
Meningiomas represent 15%-20% of all intracranial tumors. They develop from arachonoid cells of the leptomeninx and are mainly located at the level of the greater dural sinuses where the arachnoid villi are more abundant. The most involved areas are the parasaggittal regions, followed by the convexity, the sphenoid wing, the ethmoid planum, the ponto-cerebellar angle and the occipital foramen. Meningiomas can also develop in the ventricles, originating from the arachnoid cells of the choroid tela or the choroid plexuses.

The most afflicted age is between 50 and 60 years with a female/male ratio of 2:1; the higher frequency in women is due to a hormonal effect, since experimental studies have shown the presence of progesterone and estrogen receptors in meningiomas. Traumas and ionizing radiation on the skull should also be listed among the inducing causes.

Macroscopically, the meningioma appears as a globular and well-delimited mass, adherent to the dura mater and fed by meningeal vessels of the external carotid. The inferior cerebral parenchyma is compressed, at least in the typical forms, but it is not infiltrated by the neoplasia. The infiltration can involve the dural sinuses or the cranial bone.

Microscopically, the meningioma is distinguished in three histological kinds: syncytial, fibroblastic, and transitional.

Table 2.1. Intracranial tumors

Benign cerebral tumors
    Tumors of leptomeningeal origin
      Meningioma
      Hemangiopericytoma
    Nerve sheath tumors
      Neurinoma
    Vascular tumors
      Hemangioblastoma
    Dysembryogenetic tumors
      Central nervous system cysts
      Arachnoid cyst
      Epithelial cyst
      Epidermoid and dermoid cysts
      Lipoma
    Mixed cerebral tumors
      Paraganglioma
    Hypofisis adenomas
    Choroid plexus papilloma

Malignant cerebral tumors
    Astrocytoma
    Oligodendroglioma
    Ependymoma
    Medulloblastoma
    Neurocytoma
    Pineal region tumors
    Germinal cell tumors
    Chordoma
    Craniopharyngioma
    Metastases

At CT, the tumor appears isodense or hyperdense and dyshomogeneous if there are calcifications; a homogenous and intense contrast enhancement of the tumor is observed (Figs. 2.10; 2.11). This type of tumor is often associated with a zone of osseous erosion of the cranium (osteolysis) or with a support reaction (hyperostosis).

At NMR (T1-weighted images), the lesions appear hypointense compared to the cerebral parenchyma. On T2-weighted images they are homogeneously hyperintense compared to the cerebral tissue, while the calcifications appears hyperintense (Figs. 2.12-2.15). The extraparenchymal nature of the tumor is usually revealed by the presence of a liquoral halo between the tumor and the brain.

Once removed, the meningioma does not usually relapse (Fig. 2.16);

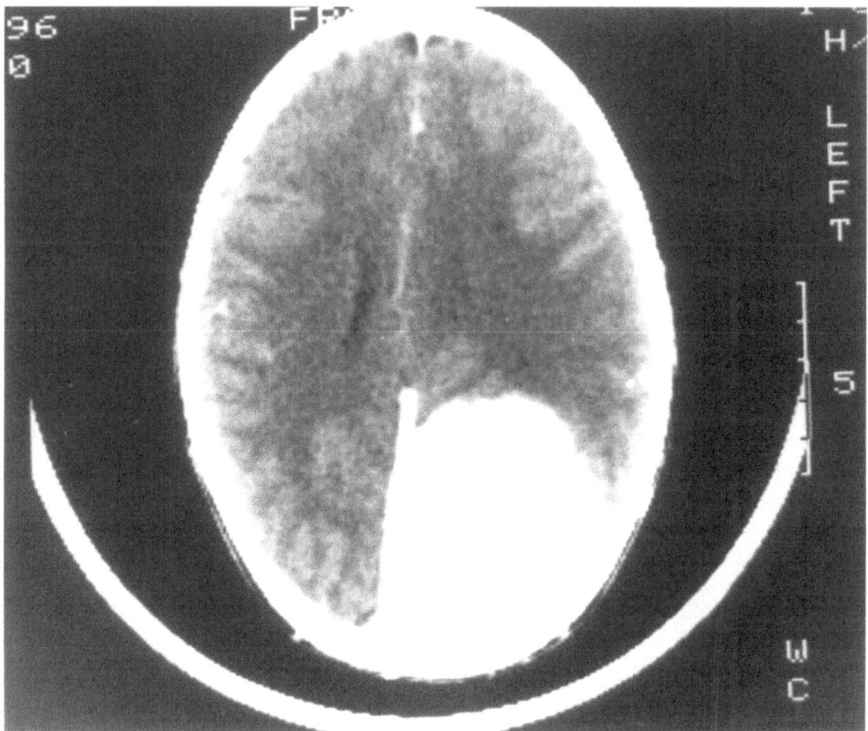

Fig. 2.10. Meningioma of the left parietal convexity. CT after contrast medium. Extensive neoformation with marked and homogeneous contrast enhancement

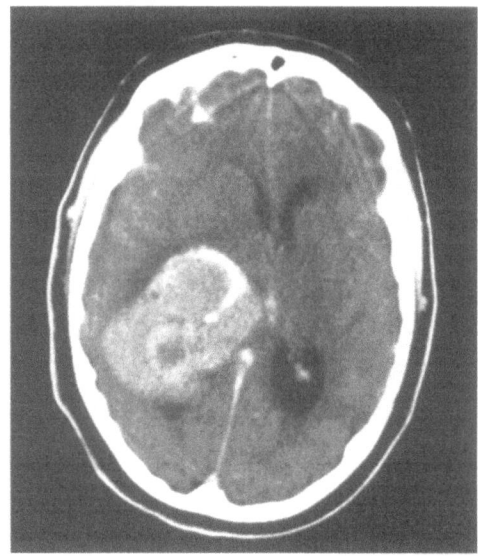

Fig. 2.11. Intraventricular meningioma. CT after contrast medium. Extensive neoformation localized inside the left ventricular trigone, with calcified nuclei and homogeneous contrast enhancement

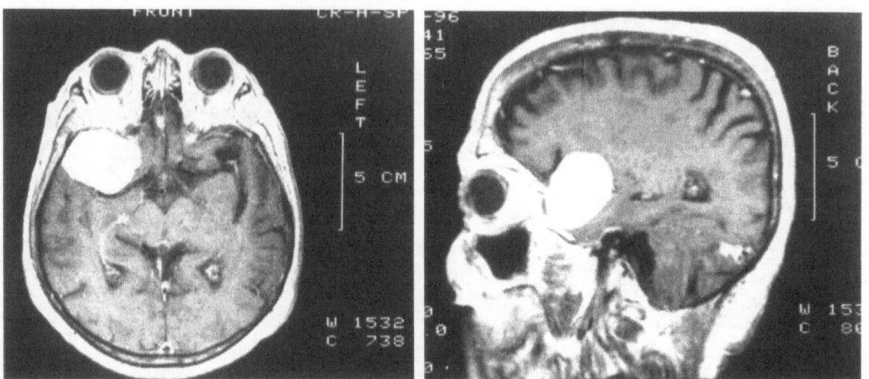

Fig. 2.12a,b. Meningioma of the middle cranial fossa. Magnetic resonance, T1-weighted images after contrast medium; axial (**a**) and sagittal (**b**) views. Neoformed pathologic and irregular roundish tissue, with marked and homogeneous contrast enhancement

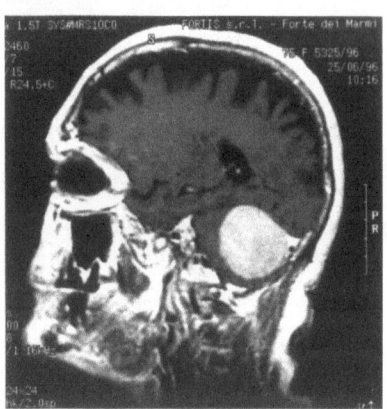

Fig. 2.13. Meningioma of the tentorium. MR, T1-weighted image, sagital view, after contrast medium. Extensive and roundish neoformation with marked and homogeneous contrast enhancement

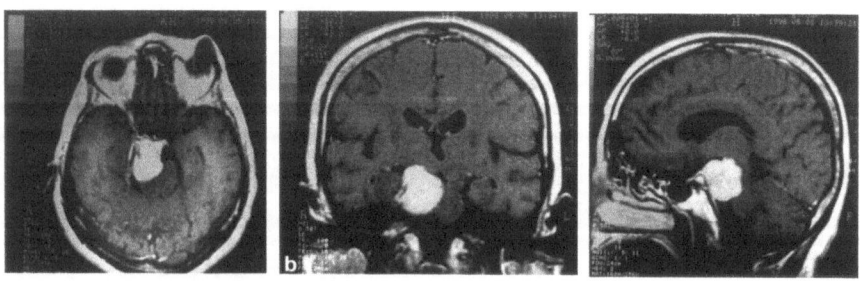

Fig. 2.14a-c. Petroclival meningioma, MR, T1-weighted images, after contrast medium; axial (**a**), coronal (**b**) and sagittal (**c**) views. Extensive neoformed pathologic tissue in the right half of the clivus and clinopetrous ligament. There is marked and homogeneous contrast enhancement and brainstem compression

Fig. 2.15. Atypical meningioma. MR, T1-weighted image, after contrast medium; sagital view. Extensive, neoformed pathologic tissue with marked contrast enhancement. Irregular and lobulated edges, expression of malignancy

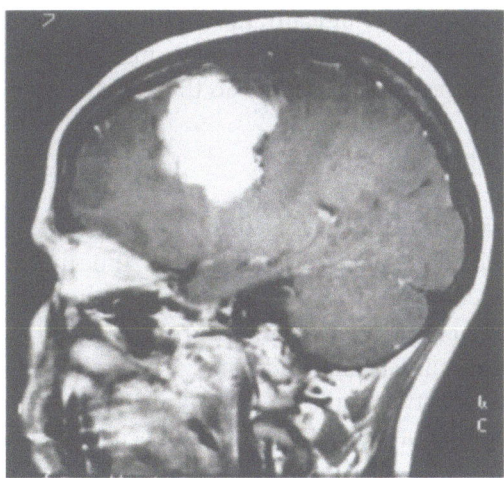

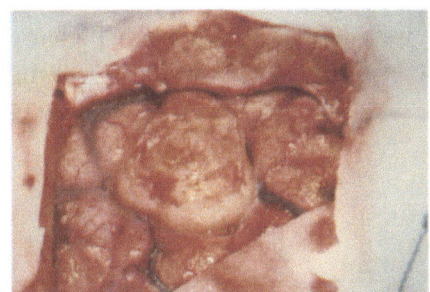

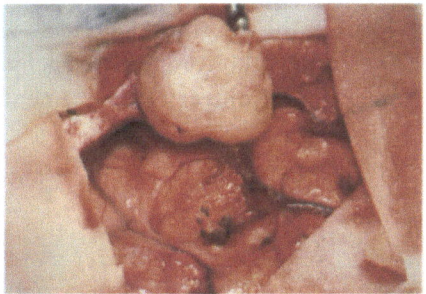

a   b

Fig. 2.16. a Intraoperative view of convexity meningioma. **b** Operative view after removal of the meningioma

however, they might if necrosis, hypercellularity, mitotic activity, cellular pleomorphism and hypervascularity are present. If the tumor cannot be completely removed, since it invades or infiltrates structures which can not be sacrified (for example the big dural venous sinuses or the internal carotid), an average recurrence in 35% of cases can be observed.

Hemangiopericytoma is thought to derive from different cell lines such as the pericytes, mesenchymal cells with contractile activity, arachnoid cells or multipotent precursor cells. Unlike meningioma, hemangiopericytoma mainly affects young males, the clinical history is shorter and there is a greater tendency to relapse even in cases of apparently complete removal.

Macroscopically, the hemangiopericytoma is a well-delimited tumor, with reddish color because of the rich vascularization and of a soft consistency. Histologically, the tumor appears highly vascularized with vessels of different caliber and many mitosis. Radiologically, the tumor presents characteristics similar to those of the meningioma.

Nerve sheath tumors

Neurinoma develops from the sheath of Schwann, and represents about 7% of all primary cerebral tumors. It occurs with irritative or specific signs of deficit at the level of the involved nerve.

Macroscopically, it appears as a solid, oval, well-delimited mass, with smooth surface and tenaciously adherent or fused to the nerve. Histologically, two kinds are distinguishable: Antoni's type A and Antoni's type B, based on the different cytological and structural components. This tumor must be distinguished from the neurofibroma that presents a more infiltrative behavior and derives mainly from small subcutaneous nerves. Neurofibroma is often associated with type I neurofibromatosis.

At CT, the neurinoma appears as a well-defined tumor, iso-hypodense compared to the cerebral parenchyma. It is often associated with a cystic component. Contrast enhancement is normally homogeneous but there

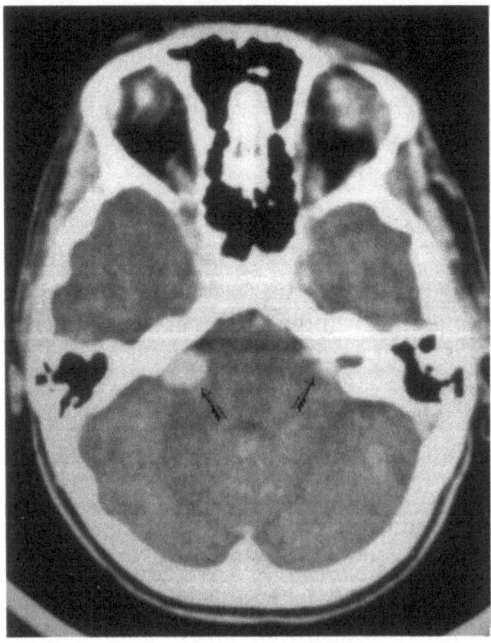

Fig. 2.17. Multiple neurinomas. CT with contrast medium. Presence of two nuclei of pathologic tissue with marked contrast enhancement. They are localized bilaterally at level of the pontocerebellar angle cisterns. Light widening of the left internal acoustic meatus

Fig. 2.18. Neurinoma of the left cranial nerve VIII. MRI, T1-weighted image after contrast medium. Pathologic tissue with marked contrast enhancement extended from the acoustic meatus to the pontocerebellar angle cistern

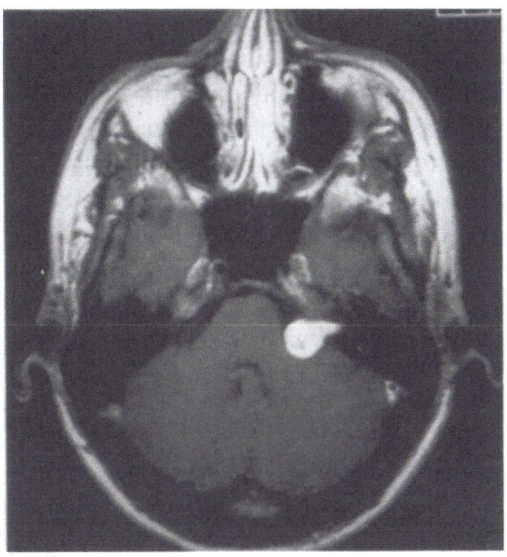

can be some zones of necrotic tissue causing a dyshomogeneous appearance (Fig. 2.17).

The neurinoma, at NMR, appears iso-hypointense in T1 and iso-hyperintense in T2. The acoustic neurinomas appear as well-defined, roundish tumors and localize at the level of and inside the acoustic meatus, which is widened as a result (Fig. 2.18).

The neurinoma is a benign tumor, must be completely removed and is not relapsing; considering that it derives from nervous tissue, it is not always possible to maintain the anatomical integrity of the affected structure.

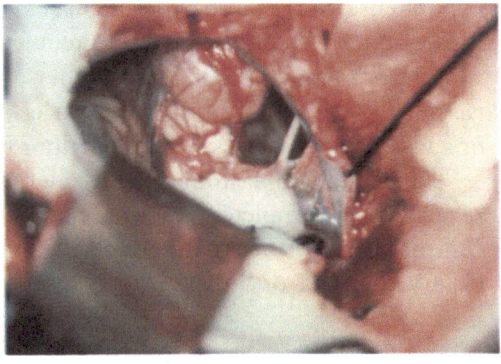

Fig. 2.19. Microsurgical aspect of a neurinoma of cranial nerve VIII

In the neurinoma of the acoustic nerve, the removal of the tumor must happen without damage the facial nerve displaced by the lesion. The surgical approach depends on the dimension of the tumor and on the extent of hypoacusis. We can perform a retromastoid suboccipital approach if the tumor is voluminous and displaces the brainstem producing a cofosis. Alternatively, we can perform a retrolabyrinthal approach if the tumor is localized inside the internal acoustic meatus, if it has a modest endocranial extension or if only hypoacusis is present (Fig. 2.19).

Vascular tumors

Hemangioblastoma constitutes 1% of intracranial tumors and 10% of posterior cranial fossa tumors. The posterior cranial fossa is the most frequent site where the hemangioblastoma tends to develop, but the cerebellar hemispheres, the vermis and the brainstem are also frequently involved.

It can occur at any age, but it is often found between the third and fifth decade of life. The lesion can be single or multiple. When multiple, it is a symptom of Von Hippel Lindow's disease and it can be associated with retinal hemangioblastomas, carcinoma of the renal cells, renal or pancreatic cysts, and pheochromocytoma.

Macroscopically, this tumor can appear either in solid or in cystic form with a small mural nodule. The solid components are reddish in color because of the vascular component, while the cystic fluid has a xanthochromic color. Microscopically, the tumor is characterized by two cellular components. The first component consists of endothelial perivascular small cells, while the second is formed by stromal cells with many vacuoles and eosinophilic granules.

CT shows either a nodular lesion or a cyst with a density similar to the cerebrospinal fluid and with a mural nodule. At NMR, the cyst appears hypointense in T1 and hyperintense in T2. Gadolinium administration causes a marked enhancement of the mural nodule (Fig. 2.20a).

Vertebral angiography shows either a vascular lesion in the form of a vascular nodule with peripheral arteries and occasional veins (Fig. 2.20b) or a wide vascular mass with anomalous ectatic vessels.

The hemangioblastoma is considered a benign tumor; it does not relapse when completely removed and is formed by a single mass. On the contrary, relapses are frequent in Von Hippel Lindau's syndrome which is observed in 15% of cases.

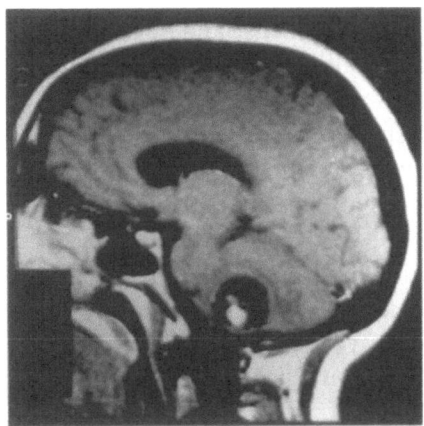 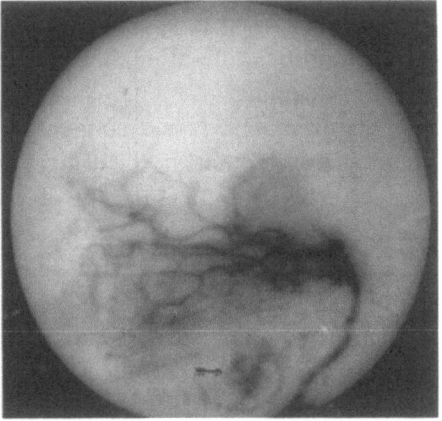

a   b

Fig. 2.20. Cerebellar hemangioblastoma. MRI, sagittal view, T1-weighted images, after contrast medium (**a**). Digital angiography of the vertebral artery (**b**). MRI shows pathologic tissue, characterized by a mural nodule with marked contrast enhancement and peripheral cystic components. Angiography shows a pathologic vascularization with supply from peripheral branches of the posterior inferior cerebellar artery

Dysembryogenetic tumors

Central nervous system cysts

Arachnoid cyst is a circumscribed accumulation of liquid similar to the cerebrospinal fluid. This cyst may or may not communicate with the subarachnoid space. The cyst can be congenital or caused by trauma or an inflammatory process.

Half of these cysts are found on the cerebral hemispheres, especially at the level of the sylvian fissure where they can be associated with a temporal lobe agenesis. In some cases they can reach considerable dimensions, compress the cerebral parenchyma and induce an intracranial hypertension syndrome. Sometimes they can be an occasional finding.

Epithelial cysts
Colloid cyst represents 1% of all intracranial tumors and derives from the invagination of a primitive ventricular cavity coated with neuroepithelium, ciliated or not.

It is a globular lesion, surrounded by a thin capsule, localized at the level of Monro's foramen. This cyst can induce an intracranial hypertension symptomatology when it obstructs, sometimes with a valve mechanism, the cerebrospinal fluid pathway.

At CT, the cyst can appear hypodense or hyperdense and does not show strong modifications after contrast medium; also at NMR it presents a large variety of signals.

Enterogenous cyst is a congenital cyst resulting from the inclusion of endodermic elements in the central nervous system. It is often observed in the vertebral column, in front of the spinal cord. It can be extradural, intradural or extramedullary.

Ependymal cyst is a cavity filled with fluid and coated with ciliated epithelium similar to ependyma. Usually, the cyst is intracerebral and it can induce intracranial hypertension or a focal syndrome when its dimensions increase due to the secreting activity of the epithelial coating.

Dermoid and epidermoid cyst are malformative cysts caused by the inclusion of a germinative layer during embryogenesis. The dermoid cyst is typically present on the midline of young patients. It is often associated with a dermic sinus and it is characterized by the inside presence of dermic elements such as sudoriparous glands, hair, and teeth. The epidermoid cyst affects elderly patients and presents a more lateral localization, mainly in the ponto-cerebellar angle. This cyst is formed by squamous and stratified

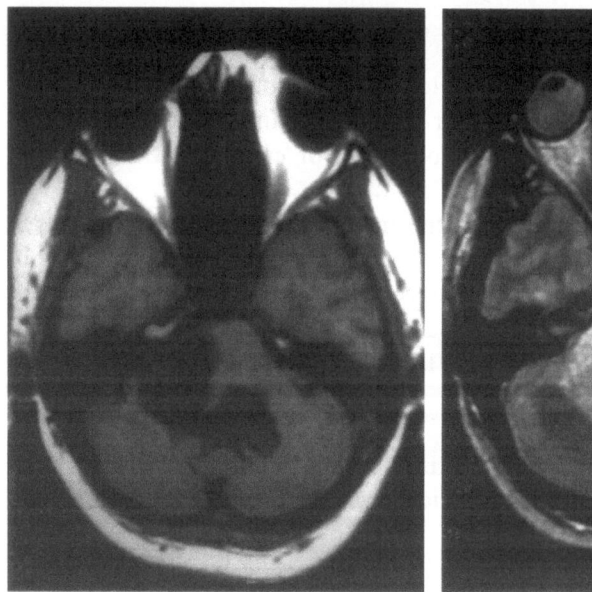 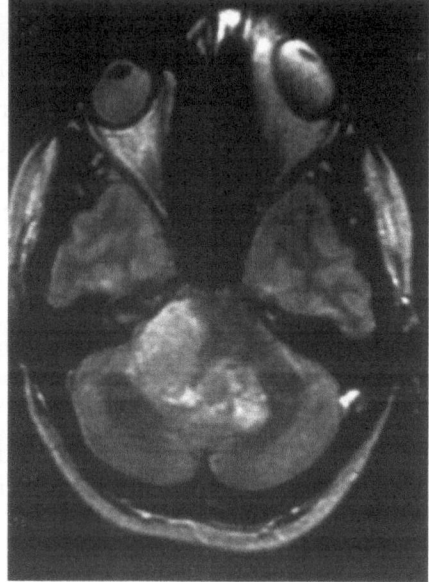

a   b

Fig. 2.21a,b. Epidermoid of the ponto-cerebellar angle. Tissue with dyshomogeneous and similar to cerebrospinal fluid intensity, localized at level of the right ponto-cerebellar angle cistern and inside the fourth ventricle

epithelium. The epidermoid cyst appears at CT as a well-delimited lesion, hypodense and without contrast enhancement. At NMR, it presents a signal similar to that of the cerebrospinal fluid (Fig. 2.21). Radiologically, the dermoid cyst presents an analogous appearance, but with a more roundish shape, sometimes with calcifications.

These dysembryogenetic tumors have a slow rate of growth and usually cause symptoms only when they have reached conspicuous dimensions. The surgical operation consists in the removal of the cystic content formed by cholesterine crystals and in the removal of the capsule, only if it has not contracted tenacious adherences with vessels and nerves. This tumor, of soft consistency, does not displace the vasculo-nervous structures, but tends to penetrate among them.

Lipoma

It is a rare, malformative, often asymptomatic tumor, even though in rare cases the patient can present epilepsy or mental retardation. The most involved areas are the corpus callosum with a partial or complete agenesis, the infundibular region, quadrigeminal lamina, and ponto-cerebellar angle.

CT shows a strongly hypodense zone which does not cause mass effect, while at NMR a characteristic hyperintensity in T1 is observed.

Hypophyseal adenomas

They are tumors derived from the adenohypophysis and represent 10% of intracranial tumors. Histological studies performed on pituitary glands obtained from autoptic material have shown the accidental presence of adenomas in 8%-23% of cases.

These benign tumors have a slow growth rate; they can be limited to the sella turcica or become extrasellar; reaching conspicuous dimensions. They can be classified into microadenomas and macroadenomas, according to their dimensions (inferior or superior to 1 cm). Another classification takes into consideration their tendency to invade adjacent structures such as cavernous sinus or sphenoid sinus; in this case they are distinguished into invasive or noninvasive adenomas. Additionally, their endocrine function can be considered, giving, to the classification a clinical character. Furthermore, the cytoplasmic staining properties can be used to distinguish the secreting or non secreting chromophobe adenomas, the ACTH-producing basophil adenomas and the GH-secreting eosinophil adenomas. With CT, the diagnosis of microadenomas is obtained with thin coronal sections which show the lesion as a hypodense zone with contrast enhancement and indirect signs, such as pituitary stalk shift or the localized erosion of the sellar floor. At NMR, they appear hypointense compared with the healthy tissue in T1; after paramagnetic contrast medium, the healthy tissue shows more contrast than the adenoma which presents a relative hypointensity (Fig. 2.22).

The radiological diagnosis of macroadenoma is easier, since this test shows a tumor raising from the sella and with super- and/or laterosellar extension. This tumor has a dyshomogeneous contrast enhancement due to possible zones of necrosis (Fig. 2.23).

The non-secreting pituitary adenomas, not susceptible to medical treatment, must be surgically removed. Although the type of surgical approach depends on the dimensions and anatomical relations with the close structures, the adenomas are treated most effectively and with fewer risks with a transphenoid microsurgical procedure. In fact, this allows a more rapid and direct approach to the hypophysis, without damaging the optic nerves and chiasm, and it is also less traumatic for the patient. On the contrary, the removal by transcranial approach is suitable when the tumor reaches the

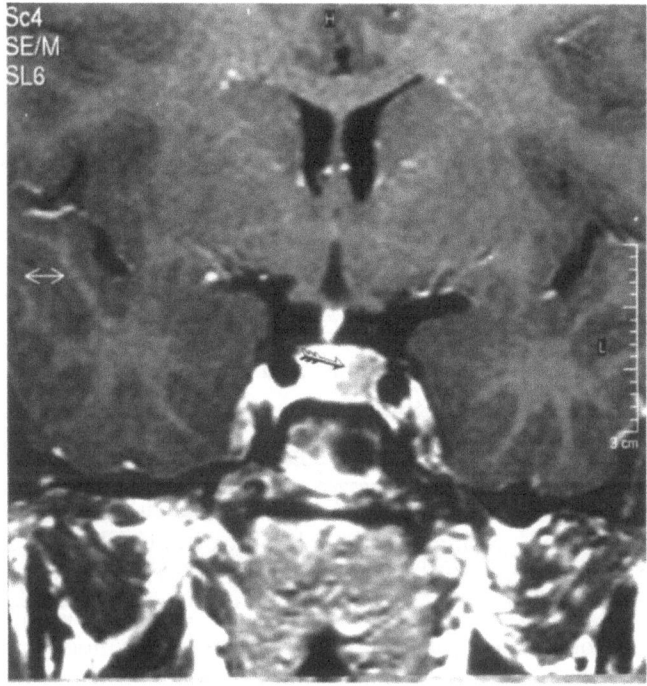

Fig. 2.22. Hypophyseal adenoma. MRI, sagital view, T1-weighted image after contrast medium. A roundish and scarcely enhancing area is localized in the left half of the pituitary gland. Displacement to the right of the pituitary stalk

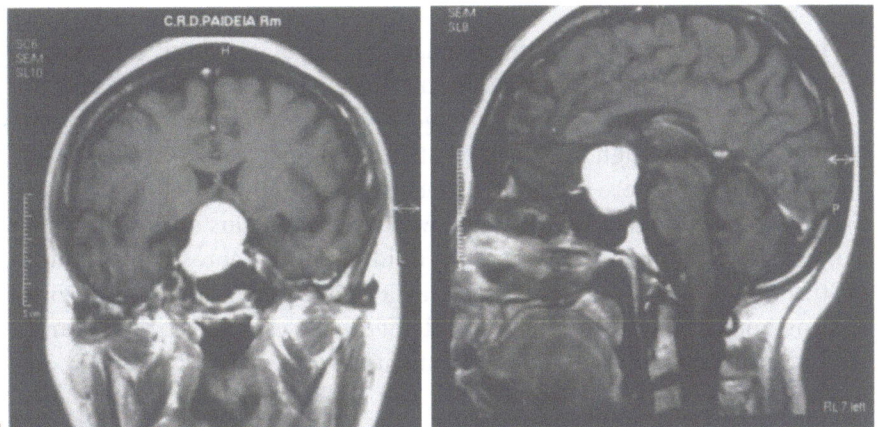

a   b

Fig. 2.23a,b. Hypophyseal macroadenoma. MRI, coronal (**a**) and sagittal (**b**) views, T1-weighted images after contrast medium. Diffuse intra-suprasellar neoformation, with compression of the optic chiasm and the third ventricle. Marked and homogeneous contrast enhancement

retrochiasmatic site, towards the anterior or middle cranial fossa (Fig. 2.24a,b).

The surgical operation is the best treatment in case of adenoma associated with acromegaly or Cushing's disease, while surgery in pituitary PRL-secreting microadenomas is still debated. In young women who want to have children, surgery is an excellent option, even if therapy with bromocryptine is possible.

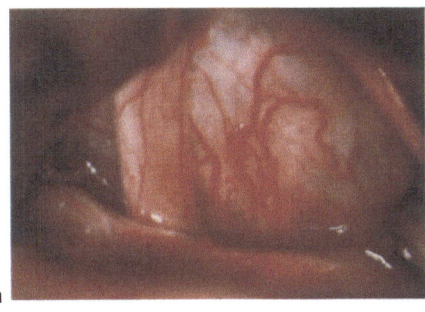
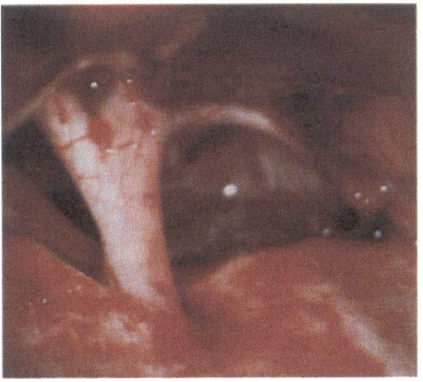

a   b

Fig. 2.24. a Microsurgical appearance of hypophyseal adenoma. **b** Microsurgical aspect after removal of the hypophyseal adenoma

Choroid plexus papilloma

This tumor derives from the neoplastic transformation of the choroid plexus epithelium and represents about 1% of all cerebral tumors and 4% of those appearing during pediatric age. This lesion can occur, in any ventricular cavity, although the fourth ventricle is more often involved; the lateral ventricles are more frequently affected in children. The choroid plexus papillomas are frequently associated with hydrocephalus caused either by a hyperproduction of cerebrospinal fluid or by cerebrospinal pathway obstruction. CT shows the neoplasia as a hypodense lesion that absorbs contrast medium and with internal calcified and cystic areas. This characteristic also explains the dyshomogeneous aspect at NMR, T1- and T2-weighted images.

Mixed cerebral tumors

Paraganglioma

The paraganglioma, or chemodectoma, originates from cells of the parasympathetic nervous system. It occurs between the fourth and fifth decade of life and it can be single or multiple. The most involved areas are the carotid artery and the glomus jugulare. In the last case, the tumor can induce a jugular foramen syndrome with paralysis of cranial nerves IX, X and XI or it can show a strong aggressivity, leading to a ponto-cerebellar angle invasion and brainstem compression. CT usually shows bone lesions and jugular foramen widening. NMR can, instead, show a characteristic, "salt and pepper" picture due to tumor vascularization and characterized by punctiform zone of void signal inside a hyperintense region.

Because of the intense vascularization, the tumor must be removed after embolization.

Malignant cerebral tumors

The concept of malignancy for all primary cerebral tumors is for some aspects different from that concerning systemic tumors. For example, the metastatic potential represents a very important prognostic factor: while the brain is a frequent site of metastasis, the primary cerebral tumors rarely metastasize outside the central nervous system. The cerebral tumor prognosis usually depends on its ability to proliferate, to determine a mass effect, to infiltrate and damage important and vital structures and, finally, to resist chemotherapy and radiotherapy. Different cell lines such as astrocytes, oligodendrocytes, and ependymal cells derive from the primary neuroectoderm. In general, with the word glioma we mean all the glial neoplasias. It must be noticed that a cerebral glioma can also be formed by the combination of two cell types.

Astrocytoma

It is a tumor in which the predominant cell line resembles the astrocyte. It represents the most frequent primary cerebral tumor and is usually divided into four histological subtypes: pilocytic, protoplasmatic, gemistocytic and fibrillary. The pilocytic astrocytoma is usually well circumscribed and presents limited zones of infiltration. It mainly occurs during pediatric age and in circumscribed zones of the cerebral parenchyma, such as the cerebellar hemisphere, the brainstem, the hypothalamus and the optic nerves and chiasm. The other subtypes appear less circumscribed, more infiltrating and have a tendency towards malignant degeneration, leading to an anaplastic astrocytoma.

The prognosis of this neoplasia is strictly connected with the involvement of vital structures, such as the brainstem, or of structures such as the language center or the motor area. The astrocytoma has been divided into four grades in relation to microscopic features such as: cytologic atypia, hypercellularity, mitotic figures, proliferation of neoformed vessels and tumoral necrosis. Therefore, we can progress from the first grade, corresponding to the so-called low grade astrocytoma, to the fourth grade corresponding to an undifferentiated tumor.

The low-grade astrocytoma infiltrates, more or less diffusely, the white substance, it does not determine a mass effect and is mainly paucisymptomatic. On the contrary, the fourth-grade neoplasia appears as an infiltrative or well-circumscribed mass, but without a cleavage plane. From the pathological point of view, it is characterized by hypercellularity, cellular and nuclear pleomorphism and the presence of mitotic figures.

At CT, the low-grade glioma appears as a hypodense area, not well defined, without perilesional edema and contrast enhancement, or as a cystic lesion with mural nodule (Fig. 2.25).

At NMR, the lesion usually appears hypointense on T1 and hyperintense on T2, and can be more or less homogeneous (Figs. 2.27-2.30).

Usually, neither CT nor MRI can define the histological grade of the glial tumor. The radiological aspect of anaplastic astrocytoma is identical to that of the glioblastoma. At CT, anaplastic astrocytoma appears as a lesion characterized by dyshomogeneous density with necrotic-cystic hypodense areas; the administration of contrast medium can cause the appearance of a peripheral edge (Fig. 2.26).

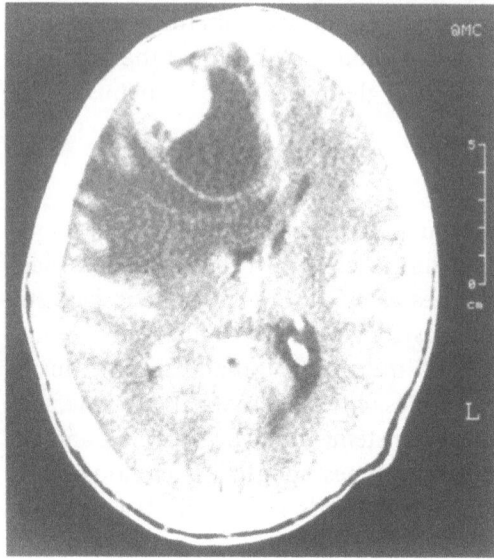

Fig. 2.25. Right frontal cystic astrocytoma. Voluminous neoformation with large cystic component and wall nodule with marked enhancement and extensive perilesional edema. Compression and displacement toward the left of the anterior part of the supratentorial ventricular system (STVS)

At NMR, a vast hetereogeneity is identifiable due to the necrosis, the hemorrhagic component and the cellularity, while the presence of serpiginous images without signal indicates the presence of neoformed vessels; in general, it is difficult to establish the limit between the tumor and the surrounding edema, usually associated with these tumors (Figs. 2.27-2.30).

Therapy for astrocytoma is surgical and the removal modality depends on its localization. The surgical operation aims at the removal of the tumor without inducing new deficits. Whenever this is not possible, a biopsy of

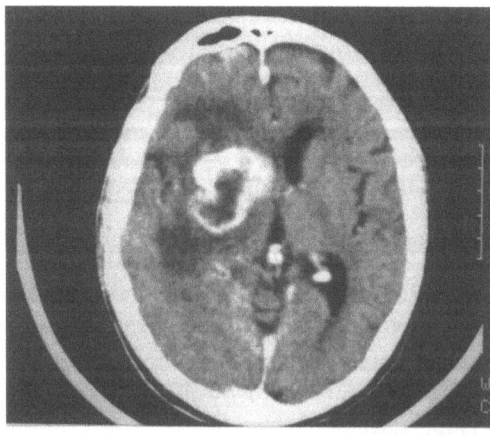

Fig. 2.26. Left frontotemporal glioblastoma. CT after contrast medium. Neoformed pathologic tissue with large zones of central necrosis, marked peripheral enhancement and extensive perilesional edema. Compression on the frontal horn of the left lateral ventricle

Fig. 2.27. Right temporo-occipital gliobastoma. MRI, T1-weighted image, axial view after contrast medium. Extensive and irregular neoformation with necrotic central zones and dyshomogeneous contrast enhancement

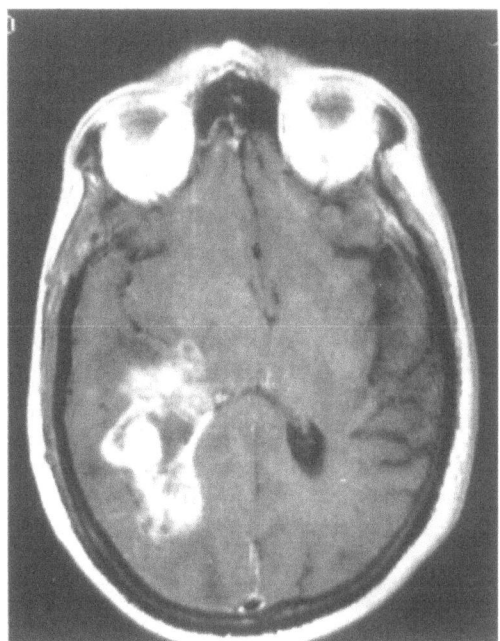

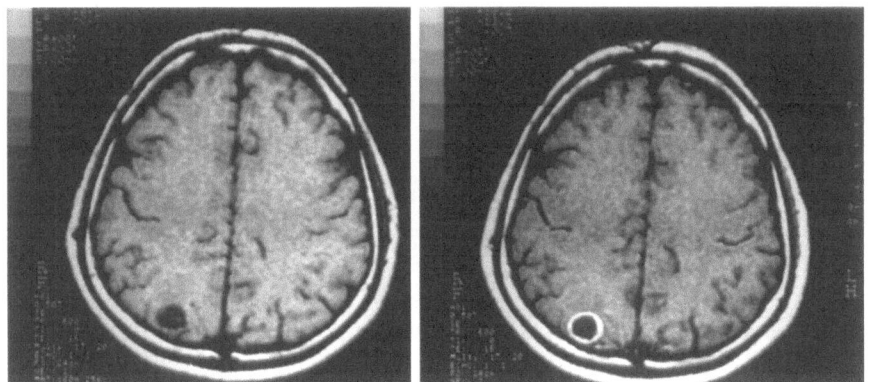

a   b

Fig. 2.28a,b. Cystic astrocytoma. Axial MRI, T1-weighted images, before (**a**) and after (**b**) contrast medium: circumscribed and pathologic tissue is located in right parietal lobe. It has a central cystic component and peripheral contrast enhancement

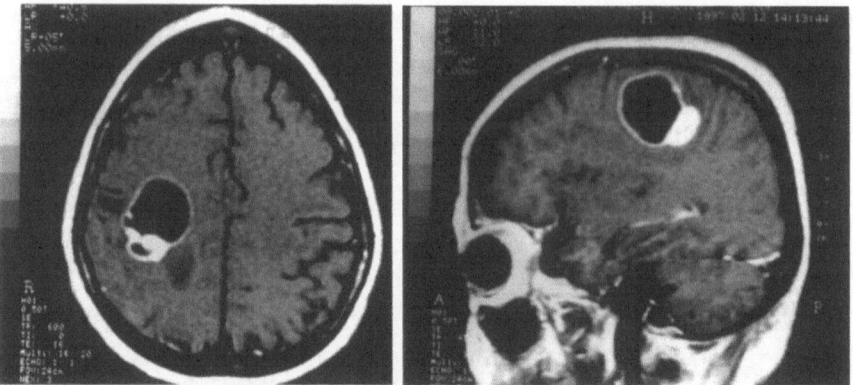

a   b

Fig. 2.29. Glioblastoma. MRI, T1-weighted images after contrast medium, axial (**a**) and sagittal (**b**) views. Extensive neoformation with central necrotic-colliquative component and peripheral solid component that presents a marked contrast enhancement

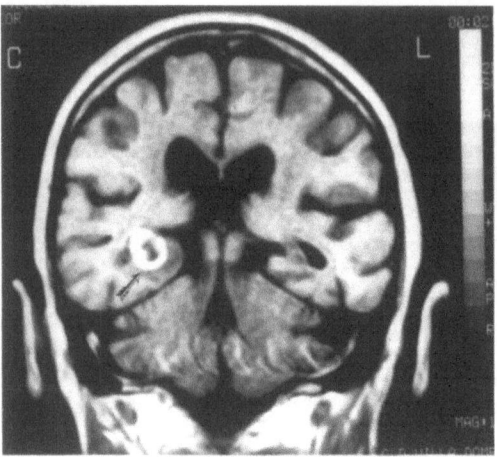

Fig. 2.30. Right hippocampal glioblastoma. MRI, T1-weighted image after contrast medium, coronal view. Right hippocampal central neoformed pathologic tissue with necrotic component and marked peripheral contrast enhancement

the lesion must be performed to evaluate the need for chemotherapy and/or radiotherapy.

Oligodendroglioma

It is a tumor formed by cells which resemble the oligodendrocytes and represents about 5% of cerebral gliomas. The most affected age is the fourth and fifth decades of life with a prevalence in men. The site most frequently involved is the white substance of the cerebral hemisphere, with tendency to invade, in advanced phases, the deep structures and the lateral ventricular walls. Usually, the patients affected by oligodendrogliomas present a long interval between the appearance of the symptoms and the diagnosis; in about 50% of cases the initial symptom is represented by an epileptic crisis.

Macroscopically, it appears as a rubbery, drab mass, with calcifications or cysts. Microscopically, the cells appear small, roundish, with black nuclei and with occasional mitosis. Foci with other glial cell types can be found. The best radiological test is NMR: the oligodendroglioma appears like a hetereogenous mass, isointense to the grey substance, with scarce edema; calcifications or microcysts can often be observed inside the tumor. Contrast enhancement is observed in 50% of cases.

Ependymoma

It represents 2%-6% of all cerebral tumors and can appear at any age but it is more frequent during childhood or adolescence. It derives from a neoplastic transformation of the ependyma, namely the epithelium coating the ventricular cavities. The tumor appears as a lobular, pinkish-gray mass protruding inside the ventricle. It often presents a clear cleavage plane. Histologically, this tumor is characterized by the presence of the perivascular pseudorosette, but numerous cytological and morphological atypias can be found.

The ependymoma is considered a malignant, slow growing tumor, with a survival period ranging from 2 to 20 years. Metastatic diffusion through the cerebrospinal canal is observed in 20% of cases.

The age at the time of diagnosis represents an important prognostic factor, since children show a lower survival rate independently of the tumor site. Furthermore, subtentorial tumors show a higher perioperative mortality and have a lower survival rate compared to the supratentorial ones. It is possible that this is due to the difficulties in completely removing a fourth ventricle ependymoma, due to the frequent involvement of the brainstem structures.

At CT, the tumor appearance is variable, usually hypodense to the basic tests and presenting a dyshomogeneous contrast enhancement (Fig. 2.31a). At NMR, it appears hypointense on T1 and hyperintense on T2 with small calcifications inside the tumor (Fig. 2.31b,c).

Medulloblastoma

It represents 1% of all primary cerebral tumors in the adult; the frequency increases to 20% in children; only 30% of these tumors affects adults. The neoplasia usually develops in the fourth ventricle and invades the cerebellum. The metastases along the cerebrospinal canal are frequent.

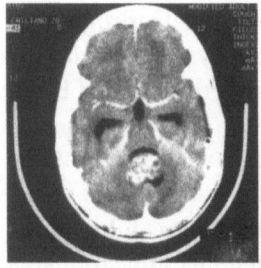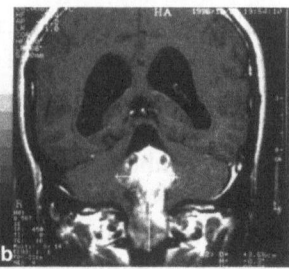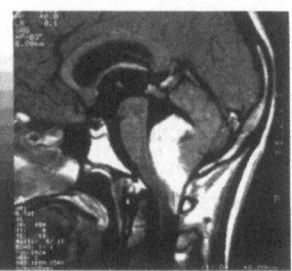

a   b   c

Fig. 2.31a-c. Ependymoma of the fourth ventricle. CT after contrast medium (a). MRI, T1-weighted images after contrast medium, coronal (b) and sagittal (c) views. Neoformed pathologic tissue localized inside the fourth ventricle with dyshomogeneous contrast enhancement. It extends downward, at level of the cisterna magna with consequent hydrocephalus

The tumor has a soft consistency and can have necrotic and hemorrhagic areas. Microscopically, it is characterized by small cells with hyperchromic and polymorphous nuclei and by numerous mitotic figures.

According to some authors, the medulloblastoma should belong to the primary neuroectoderm tumors, a group of embryonic tumors that includes neuroblastoma, ependymoblastoma, and pinealoblastoma.

At CT, the tumor appears like a solid mass, slightly hyperdense with homogeneous and intense contrast enhancement.

At NMR, the lesion is isointense to the cerebellar parenchyma, both on T1 and on T2 sequences, due to its high cellularity. A more or less marked enhancement is observed after gadolinium.

In the case of metastases along the cerebrospinal canal, it is recommendable to administer a chemotherapeutic treatment before proceeding to the surgical operation. After the surgical removal, it is appropriate to perform radiation therapy on the tumor site and on the whole neuraxis.

Neurocytoma

The neurocytoma has been only recently recognized as a distinct pathological lesion. It is a tumor of neuronal origin presenting an intermediate grade of differentiation between the cerebral neuroblastoma and the gangliocytoma. This tumor is found in young adults and presents a conspicuous intraventricular component since it often develops on the midline at the level of the transparent septum. The neurocytoma is rarely invasive, but the complete removal results, at time, difficult. It is considered a slow growing tumor. Its prognosis is not well known yet, being quite infrequent and of recent definition (Fig. 2.32a,b).

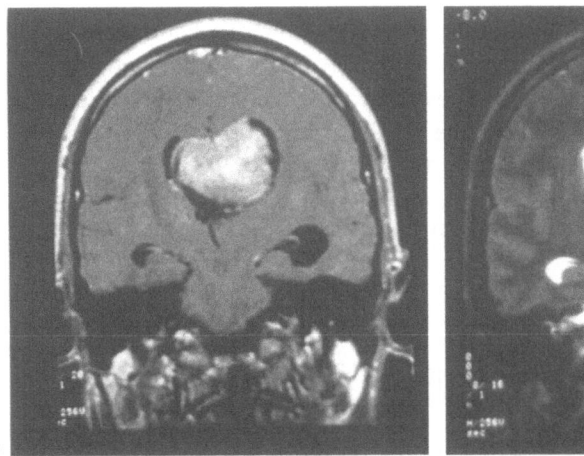
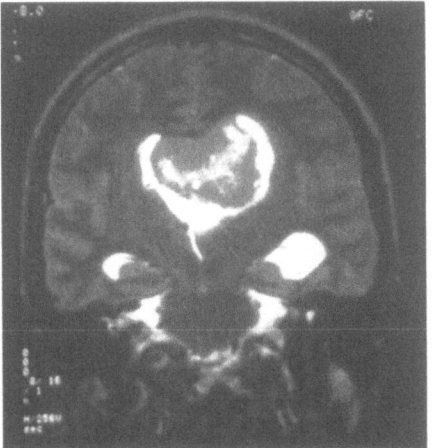

a   b

Fig. 2.32a,b. Central neurocytoma. MRI, coronal views, T1-weighted image after contrast medium (**a**) and T2-weighted image (**b**). Extensive pathologic tissue, localized inside the STVS which presents a dyshomogeneous contrast enhancement and hyperintense zones on the T2-weighted image due to cystic degeneration

Pineal region tumors

They represent little more than 1% of cerebral tumors in the adult and arise from the neoplastic transformation of developing or mature pinealocytes. Hence primary neoplasias, such as the pinealoblastoma, or differentiated lesions, like the pinealocytoma, can be found (Fig. 2.33).

The pinealoblastoma appears more frequently during the first decade of life, while the pinealocytoma is more often found in young adults. These

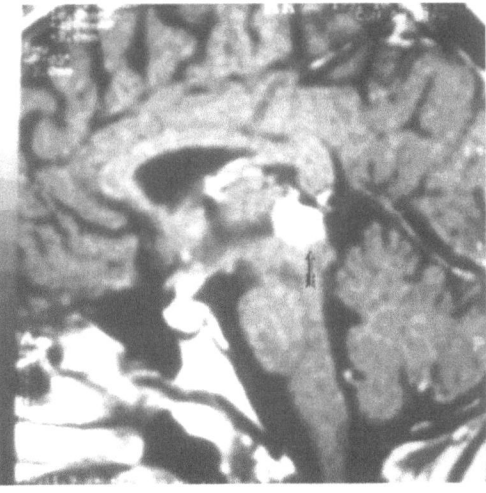

Fig. 2.33. Pinealoblastoma. MRI, sagittal view, T1-weighted images, after contrast medium. Pathologic tissue with a marked and homogeneous contrast enhancement, localized at the level of the pineal gland. There is another nucleus of pathologic tissue localized at the level of the proximal part of the pituitary stalk which is expression of metastasis along the cerebrospinal pathway

neoplasias tend to compress and invade the quadrigeminal lamina colliculi and sylvian aqueduct. Their prognosis is strictly linked to their tendency to disseminate neoplastic cells along the cerebrospinal canal. This tendency is inversely proportional to their grade of differentiation and explains why craniospinal radiotherapy is ideal for these tumors.

A patient affected by pinealoblastoma rarely survives over two years, while the prognosis of patients affected by pinealocytoma is more promising.

Germinal cells tumors

They are relatively rare tumors, representing less than 1% of all cerebral tumors. They develop on the midline at the level of the pineal region and in suprasellar areas. In this group we can distinguish: germinoma, teratoma (they represent respectively 60% and 20% of the germinal cells tumors), and the more infrequent embryonal carcinoma and choriocarcinoma.

The symptomatology is due to triventricular hydrocephalus caused by obstruction of the sylvian aqueduct (when the pineal region is involved) or to disorders of the hypothalamic-pituitary axis.

The prognosis depends on the cellular type; the immature teratoma is the most highly malignant. The finding of neoplastic dissemination along the cerebrospinal canal is frequent. Some of these tumors tend to be well-circumscribed; others, like the germinoma, have an infiltrative nature, making their complete removal impossible and highly risky. Fortunately, they are highly sensitive to radiation therapy. These tumors present hormonal activity and their secreted products can be found in the blood and in the cerebrospinal fluid. Elevated blood or CSF levels of human chronic gonadotropin (HCG) are found in the choriocarcinoma; teratoma tends to produce carcinoembryonic antigen (CEA), while the germinoma is not associated with the production of any particular hormone, even if an increase in HCG can be occasionally found.

Chordoma

It is a low grade malignant tumor derived from residues of the notochord, most frequently found in the sacral region. Forty percent of these tumors are found on the midline, at the level of the clivus and they rarely metastasize (on the contrary, sacral chordomas are highly metastatic). It is a neoplasia that infiltrates and destroys bones and soft tissues, while the invasion of the cerebral parenchyma is rare; the brainstem is compressed by the tumor through the dura mater. Its infiltrative character and its localization on the midline make its complete removal difficult. The average survival time is about 5-7 years.

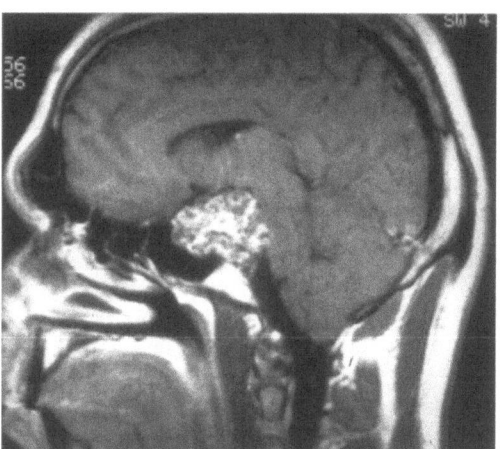

Fig. 2.34. Chordoma of the clivus. MRI, sagittal view, T1-weighted image. Extensive and dyshomogeneously hyperintense pathologic tissue on T1-weighted images. It is localized in the clivus and has an anterior extension at level of the sphenoid sinus and a posterior tip on the ventral surface of the brainstem

At CT, it appears as a well delimited tumor with intratumoral calcifications, presenting a more or less intense contrast enhancement.

At NMR, the chordoma appears hypointense on T1 and hyperintense on T2; the signal is often dyshomogeneous because of past hemorrhage and calcifications (Fig. 2.34).

Craniopharyngioma

It is a rare neoplasia of the cranial base arising from the sella turcica; it represents 2%-3% of all cerebral tumors, with greater incidence in children and adolescents. The cellular origin of this tumor is still debated. One possibility is that it derives from the squamous epithelium of Ratchke's pouch, at the level of the pituitary stalk. The craniopharyngioma is considered a slow growing, benign tumor, however, the surgical removal is difficult since it tends to infiltrate the nearby structures (cerebral parenchyma, cranial nerves and blood vessels). With plain radiography, it is possible to observe a widening of the sellar aditus with suprasellar calcifications. At CT, the appearance is dyshomogeneous because of the calcifications associated with the cystic components. At NMR, the signal coming from the cyst content is variable, depending on the concentrations of proteins, cholesterine, and methemoglobin (Fig. 2.35a,b).

Metastases

The tumors that most frequently cause cerebral metastases are the adenocarcinoma, the "small cell" lung carcinoma, breast carcinoma, non Hodgkin's lymphoma and melanoma. The metastatic invasion occurs through the blood stream (neoplastic embolism) and often the cerebral

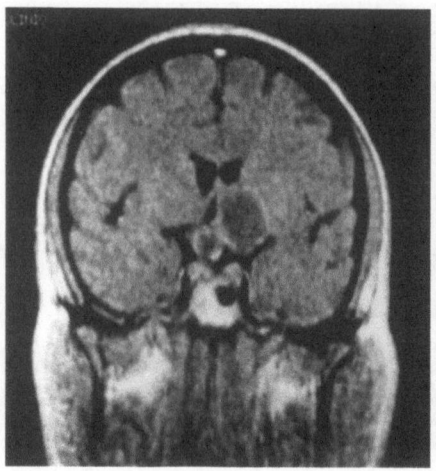
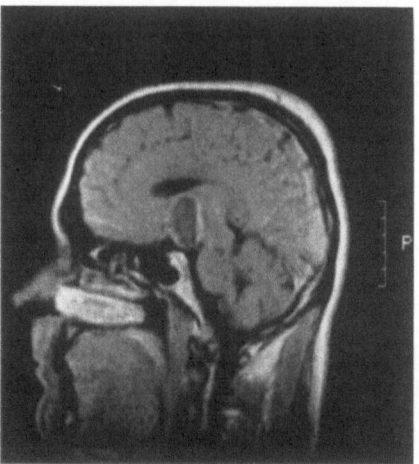

a

b

Fig. 2.35a,b. Craniopharyngioma. MRI, T1-weighted images, coronal (**a**) and sagittal (**b**) views. The solid component of the pathologic tissue is located in intrasellar zone and the cystic component tissue is located in suprasellar zone

localization represents the initial symptom of a neoplasia. 30% of patients affected by carcinoma present a cerebral metastasis, mainly found in the supratentorial area. NMR with gadolinium represents the best test for the radiological diagnosis, since it is more sensitive than CT. The lesions can be hypointense or isointense compared to the cerebral parenchyma and are surrounded by a remarkable perilesional edema affecting the white substance. Paramagnetic contrast medium administration is fundamental because it emphasites the presence of small cortical lesions with no edema (Fig. 2.36).

The surgical removal is indicated only if a single lesion is present. A regression of the cerebral edema and an improvement of the neurogical conditions follow the complete removal of the tumor.

Therapy

The treatment of cerebral tumors can be surgical, radiotherapeutic and chemotherapeutic.

The best choice of treatment is achieved analyzing different factors: first of all the histological nature of the lesion, then the localization, the dimensions of the tumor and the age of the patient. Usually, the first-choice treatment is the surgical operation with the total, when possible, or partial removal of the tumor, in order to stop or delay the appearance of neuro-

Fig. 2.36. Cerebellar metastases. MRI, T1-weighted image, coronal view after contrast medium. Multiple nuclei of neoformed pathologic tissue with variable dimensions and morphology and marked contrast enhancement

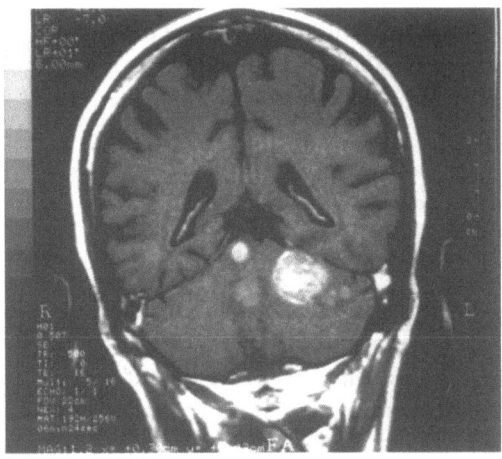

logical deficits and intracranial hypertension. All the benign tumors (meningiomas (Fig. 2.16), neurinomas (Fig. 2.19), adenomas (Fig. 2.24), craniopharyngiomas, epidermoid and dermoid cysts) must be radically removed, together with the malignant ones (gliomas, ependymomas, oligo-dendrogliomas, metastases) not localized in critical regions. When the tumor is localized in a critical region (motor and sensory areas, diencephalo-hypothalamic area, basal nuclei, brainstem), the removal must be cautious and limited to a simple biopsy, allowing a decompression without provoking more serious neurological deficits.

The postoperative survival period depends on the nature of the tumor and the extent of the removal. When a benign tumor is completely removed, total recovery is definitive. The most immature glial tumors with a high grade of cellularity (glioblastoma, grade III glioma, ependymoblastoma) most likely relapse within 8-14 months, even though radio- and chemotherapy have been administred and the patient has led a normal life for some months after the operation. The gliomas with a lower grade of cellularity show various behaviors: in average, they relapse within 2-3 years. In case of oligodendrogliomas, there are more chances of a longer survival.

Radiotherapy and chemotherapy are complementary to the surgical treatment. Radio- and chemotherapy aim to interfere with the metabolism of the neoplastic cells. The drugs, once penetrated into the tumor cells, interfere with their cellular functions and lead to death. Radiotherapy, using ionizing radiation, reaches the tumoral target cells causing the destruction of the biochemical unit of the cell.

It is to be noted that radiotherapy and chemotherapy increase very little the survival time in case of immature gliomas and metastases. On the

contrary, medulloblastomas, ependymomas of the fourth ventricle and germinomas show a clear improvement in the prognosis, with an average survival time of 8-10 years.

Pseudotumor cerebri

Pseudotumor cerebri is an intracranial hypertension syndrome not caused
by a tumor or hydrocephalus. This disease is more frequent in women,
especially if obese or pregnant. It is mainly associated with hematologic-
endocrine diseases (Addison's disease) or conditions which block the
venous reflux, such as cardiac congenital malformations, dural sinus
thrombosis, pulmonary diseases with venous hypertension, as well as
many hypo- and hypervitaminoses or rapid suspension of corticosteroid
treatment.

The formation of cerebral edema due to this disease is of uncertain origin. It may be related to high levels of vasopressin in the cerebrospinal
fluid, which may contribute to water accumulation in the tissue.

The clinical picture shows symptoms and signs of slight intracranial
hypertension, but papillary stasis is a consistent finding. The characteristic
evolution leads, almost spontaneously, to a complete recovery after a symptomatic therapy based on osmotic diuretics and cortisone. Repeated evac-
uative rachicentesis is also effective. In the malignant form, with a more or
less fast evolution, a bilateral temporal decompression is necessary.

Phacomatosis

They include hamartomatous malformations involving the nervous system, the skin, the eyes, and the vascular system. They do not always require
surgical operation but they are usually kept under constant observation by
a neurosurgeon.

Von Recklinghausen's neurofibromatosis

This is a hereditary disease with autosomal dominant character. It is
characterized by "milk and coffee" spots on the skin, and neurofibromas
involving cutaneous and deep nerves, roots, visceral nerves and pigmenta-
tion of the iris (Fish's nodules or pigmented hamartomas of the iris, with
high incidence).

Clinically, the symptoms and signs associated with the dermal lesions
are various: a) macrocephaly, not connected with hydrocephalus or tumor;

b) frequent convulsive crises even in absence of tumoral masses; c) headache, sometimes with migrainous features; d) ischemic and ictal episodes, due to compression of the main arteries; e) arterial hypertension, caused by damage to the renal arteries or due to a pheochromocytoma; f) different levels of mental retardation; and g) itch induced by histamine produced by the mastocytes of the neurofibromas. Moreover, optic nerve or chiasm glioma, palpebral swelling, intraorbital meningioma (relatively more frequent in subjects with neurofibromatosis and with constant exophthalmos) have been observed. Visceral neurofibromatosis causes symptoms and signs relative to the organ involved. In presence of functional deficits, a surgical treatment is essential.

Tuberous sclerosis

Usually, this is a hereditary disease with autosomal dominant character. It is characterized by neurological, cutaneous and ocular manifestations and affects males and females. In 20%-30% of cases, the diagnosis is possible before the second year of age.

The anatomical characteristics of this neurological disorder are: sclerous areas and tubers, diffuse fibrillary gliosis, and gigantocellular subependymal astrocytomas, which represent the most typical feature of the disease.

Clinically, the neurological lesions provoke epileptic crises of the "grand mal epilepsy" type. In children, neck, trunk, and limb spasms are present instead. Choreic movements are another possible manifestation.

Electroencephalography shows slow waves and peaks. Sometimes there is intracranial hypertension; mental retardation is also frequent. The cutaneous lesions are mainly represented by sebaceous adenomas and "mountain ash leaf" spots.

The ocular manifestations are astrocytic hamartomas of the retina. Visceral lesions can also be found in this disease, such as renal angiomyolipoma, cardiac rhabdomyoma and pulmonary pleural cyst. Surgical therapy is applied only in case of symptomatic subependymal astrocytomas, which are not sensitive to radiotherapy.

Von Hippel-Lindau disease

This is a hereditary disease, autosomal dominant, characterized by the coexistence of capillary angioma of the retina and cerebellar hemangioma, associated with cystic tumors of the pancreas, kidney, and epididymous. Sometimes syringomyelic cavities develop.

Clinically, this disease occurs during the second or third decade of life. Symptomatology depends on the different localization of the lesions, but

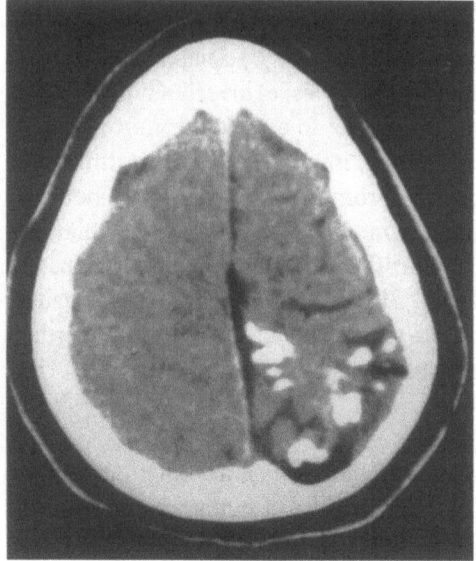

Fig. 2.37. Sturge-Weber malformation. Cerebral CT. Multiple cortical calcifications associated with a sectorial dilatation of the subarachnoid spaces

intracranial hypertension seems to prevail, especially when the vermis cerebelli is involved, with early obstruction of cerebrospinal fluid flow. Today, the diagnosis is facilitated by neuroimaging. The therapy is surgical and aims at the removal of the hemangioma. When necessary, retinal angiomas can be photocoagulated.

Encephalotrigeminal angiomatosis (or Sturge-Weber syndrome)

This is characterized by an encephalomeningeal angioma associated with facial angioma. Other symptoms can be partial epileptic crises, intracranial calcifications, and hypsilateral glaucoma.

The facial angioma, already present at birth, involves all the homolateral trigeminal territory or one of its branchs; it is also called nevus flammeus (port-wine stain) and is formed by dilated capillaries.

The encephalomeningeal angioma is formed by numerous aneurysmal dilations, which deepen into the cerebral parenchyma from the meningeal sheaths (Fig. 2.37).

The symptomatology is various: epileptic crises, often partial ones, homonymous lateral hemianopsia. Intracranial hypertension is rare. Sometimes glaucoma and buphthalmos are present homolaterally to the facial angioma.

The diagnosis is easy but the prognosis is inauspicious. No radical therapy is possible.

3. Intracranial aneurysms

The arterial aneurysm is a circumscribed or diffuse dilation of an intracranial artery segment. According to their morphology, we distinguish the aneurysms into: saccular, fusiform, and dissecting.

The most frequent variety is the saccular or vestigial, representing about 95% of cases. It consists of a roundish or oval sac with a fundus (its apex is called "dome") and with a neck which indicates the insertion point into the artery. Sometimes the neck is not present and the whole sac arises from the artery.

Epidemiology

According to an extrapolation of various autopsical reports, the incidence of intracranial arterial aneurysm, even if very variable in relation to the different ethnic groups, is about 5% in the adult American and European populations. Hemorrhages due to the breaking of an aneurysm affect 6-10/ 100 000 individuals every year. Unfortunately, only less than 40% of the patients will have a functionally normal life afterwards. It has been demonstrated that about 2% of the whole population carries a cerebral aneurysm, which will break in 1% of cases, causing death in about 0. 5% of them.

Etiopathogenesis

The physiopathology of aneurysmatic sac formation is still debated. The most valued etiopathogenetic hypotheses are the dysembryogenetic theory and the acquired theory.

The dysembryogenetic theory, formulated by Eppinger in 1887 and then supported by Forbus and Brener, explains aneurysm formation with a defective development of the tunica media and inner elastic coating of the vasal wall during embryogenesis, mainly at the level of the arterial bifurcations (Fig. 3.1). Elements in favor of this hypothesis are: a) the association of the aneurysm with other cerebral malformations, aorta coarctation, polycystic kidney, extracranial muscular fibrous dysplasia, Marfan's syndrome, tuberous sclerosis, or Ehlers-Danlos' syndrome; b) the prevailing localization of aneurysms at the level of Willis' circle areas, which undergo important modifications during embryonic life in order to achieve the final vasal circuitry of the foetus; and c) arterial aneurysms occuring during pediatric age and in middle-aged patients whose arterial trees are free from arteriosclerotical foetus alternations.

The acquired hypothesis explains the formation of the aneurysm by taking into consideration the degenerative or destructive events that can cause thinning and weakening of the vasal wall. The most frequent are: a) arteriosclerosis, b) bacterial, mycotic and neoplastic emboli; c) trauma; and d) systemic diseases involving the blood vessels (e.g. lupus erythematosus, Moya-Moya disease, granulomatous angitis).

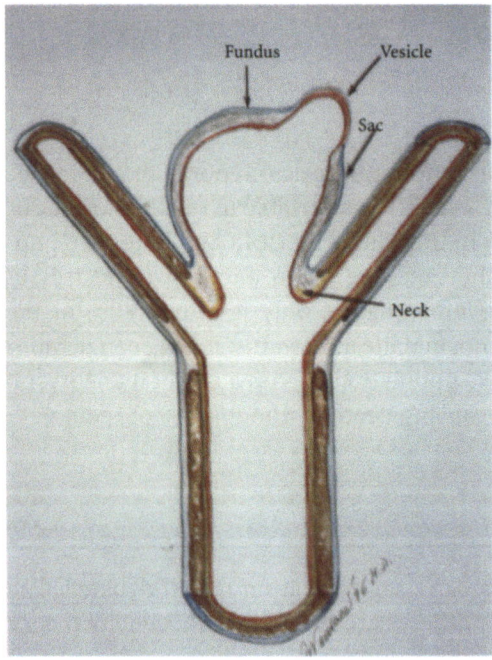

Fig. 3.1. Aneurysmatic sac formation

It is likely that intracranial aneurysms have a multifactorial etiopathogenesis. Predisposing congenital factors can sum with local and/or systemic factors to cause a further weakening of the arterial wall. Under hemodynamic stress, the compromised vessel undergoes an ectatic dilation.

Other important factors for the formation and rupture of the aneurysmatic sac are: arterial hypertension, especially gestational hypertension, use of tobacco or alcohol, and prolonged use of analgesic drugs. The practice of intense physical acivity does not seem to be instrumental to breaking an aneurysm because 30%-40% of the bleedings occur at rest.

The probability of an aneurysm breaking increases gradually with age, reaching its apex during the sixth decade of life. It should be noted that aneurysms are more prevalent in women (55%-58%). The most frequently affected arteries are: anterior communicating artery (38%-40%), internal carotid artery (31%-33%), middle cerebral artery (17%-20%) and the vertebro-basilar group (8%-10%). Intracranial aneurysms can be single or multiple (15%-20%), and have a familial incidence of about 10%.

In relation to their dimensions, they are called "baby aneurysms" if the largest diameter of the sac is less than 5 mm, "small aneurysms" if it is between 5 and 12 mm, "large aneurysms" between 12 and 25 mm, and "giant aneurysms" over 25 mm.

Symptomatology

The symptomatology of cerebral aneurysms varies according to the localization, dimensions and to the probability of the sac breaking. It is possible to distinguish two clinical kinds: a) hemorrhagic and b) pseudotumoral.

Hemorrhagic symptomatology

The most frequent onset of the intracranial aneurysms is certainly the subarachnoid hemorrhage (SAH), even though the hemorrhage can involve the cerebral parenchyma and the ventricular system.

The diagnosis is easy when SAH occurs in a typical way: e.g. a patient of about 50 years of age, who feels strong occipito-nuchal headache, described as a dagger blow to the nape, with vomit, transient loss of consciousness, neck stiffness, increase in temperature and diffuse retinal hemorrhages. Unfortunately, in many patients SAH causes a cascade of events that are often fatal, independently of a further bleeding.

In 25%-50% of cases, the neurological picture described is preceded, during the days or weeks before the SAH, by "minor leaks" or "warning leaks". These early symptoms could be considered as an early syndrome, certainly not typical. The early symptoms are: light headache or light and continuous nuchal pain (often erroneously abscribed to cervical arthrosis), increase in temperature (37.2°-37.8° C), retrorbital pain or paresthesias and facial pains, diplopia, decrease in vision or other aspecific symptoms.

The "warning leaks" are the expression of small subarachnoid bleedings or of an increase or distension of the aneurysmatic sac. A manifest SAH generally occurs after a varying and unpredictable number of these warning signs, with a more or less catastrophic clinical picture.

The neurological examination is essential to evaluate the patient from a diagnostic and therapeutic point of view. In the past years, various scales of evaluation have been proposed, but the most used is Hunt and Hess' scale.

In Hunt and Hess' scale, patients affected by SAH are classified into five grades of severity: 0 = asymptomatic; I = headache or light neck stifness; II = headache and strong neck stiffness; III = more or less severe neurological deficits; IV = consciousness alteration with or without connected deficits; and V = areflexic coma. Morbidity and mortality increase with the increasing grade in which the patient is placed.

For a suitable treatment of SAH, it is necessary to know the clinical history and the most common consequences.

In patients surviving the first hemorrhage, the highest risk of rebleeding is during the first 48 hours. During the first day, the probability that the aneurysm will bleed again is about 4% and it progressively decreases, so that on the third day the risk is down to 1.5%. Therefore, 14 days after SAH, the cumulative risk of rebleeding is of about 19%-20%; after six months it is about 50%. One of the most frequent and most serious complications of SAH is cerebral ischemia caused by vasospasm, which generally starts after 7-10 days. Vasospasm is the principal cause of death and disability after SAH (14% of cases versus 7% of the bleeding).

The risk of symptomatic vasospasm can be evaluated from the first cerebral CT: when a thick hematic accumulation is observed in the subarachnoid cisterns (mainly at the perimesencephalic level), the risk of vasospasm is higher compared to patients with a thinner one.

Communicating or not-communicating hydrocephalus is another common consequence of SAH. In 10% of cases, it requires an internal shunt of the cerebrospinal fluid.

Pseudotumoral symptomatology
Intracranial aneurysms can slowly increase in volume with time, reaching conspicuous dimensions and causing mass-effect symptoms on the compressed or displaced neurovascular structures or symptoms of intracranial

hypertension.

The onset of paralysis of cranial nerve III is typical. It is the sign of a carotid aneurysm at the level of the posterior communicating artery, posterior cerebral artery or distal part of the basilar artery.

Diagnostic iter

The diagnostic protocol for a patient affected by SAH starts with CT without contrast medium. During the first days after the hemorrhage, CT shows, in over 95% of cases, blood in the subarachnoid spaces, sometimes at intraventricular-intraparenchymal levels and possibly in the subdural space.

Currently, CT (Fig. 3.2) is still more dependable than NMR for the diagnosis of SAH, while NMR and especially angio-NMR, is more sensitive than CT in showing the presence of an aneurysmatic sac (Fig. 3.3). If CT is negative, but the clinical picture is extremely suggestive of a SAH, a lumbar puncture can be suitable for searching potential traces of blood in the cerebrospinal fluid.

The dignostic *iter* must always be completed with a panangiogram of the cerebral vessels, which can show one or more aneurysms (multiple in the 15% of cases), the artery of origin, the direction, the sac and neck dimensions, other associated vascular malformations, and the possible presence of vasospasm (Figg. 3.4; 3.5).

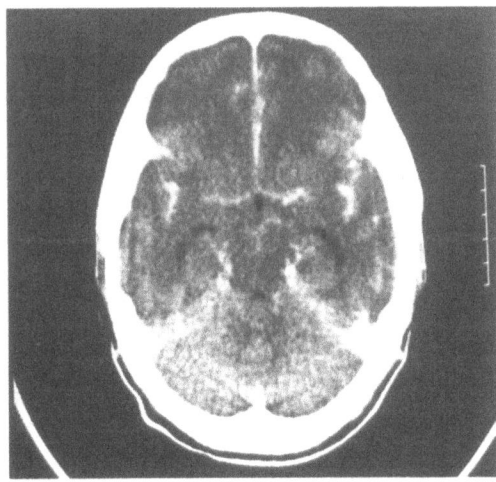

Fig. 3.2. Subarachnoid hemorrhage. Cerebral CT. Hematic hyperdensity localized at the level of the basal subarachnoid spaces

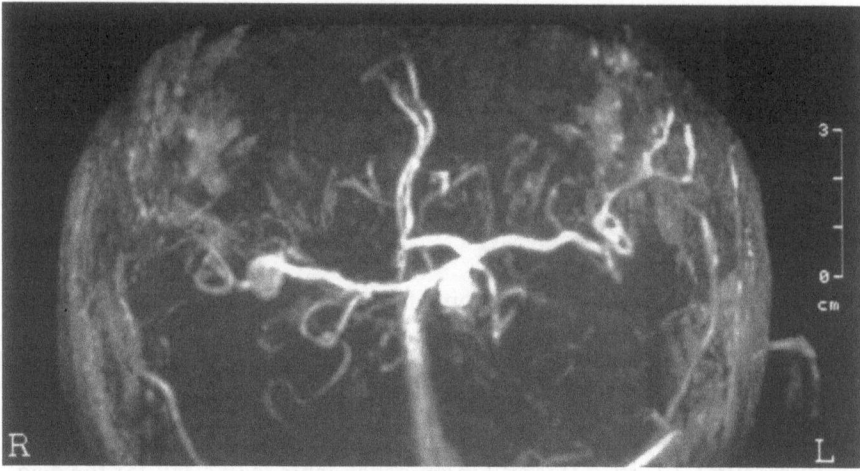

Fig. 3.3. Multiple aneurysms. Cerebral angio NMR. Presence of two aneurysmatic dilations the most voluminous is localized at the level of the left communicating posteriorcarotid and the other is localized at the level of the right middle cerebral artery bifurcation

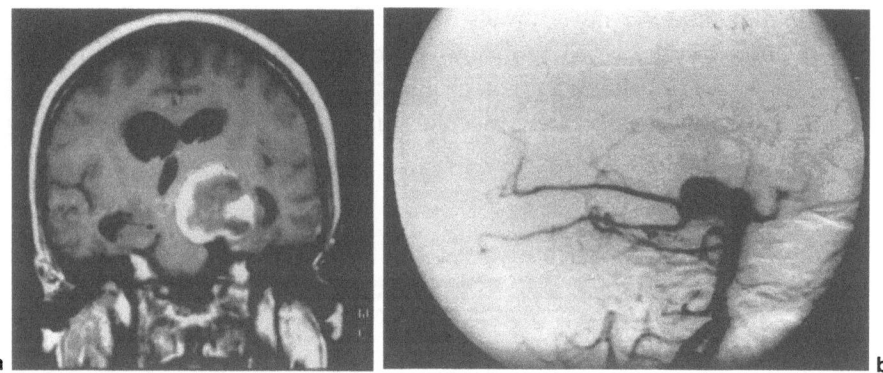

Fig. 3.4. Giant aneurysm of the right cerebral posterior artery. **a** NMR, T1-weighted, coronal view. **b** Arterial digital angiography of the basilar-vertebral tract

General strategies of treatment

To plan a suitable medical and surgical treatment of SAH due to the rupture of an intracranial aneurysm, it is first of all necessary to examine the patient carefully, using Hunt and Hess' scale. Considering that the highest incidence of rebleeding is within the first 48 hours after SAH, the best ther-

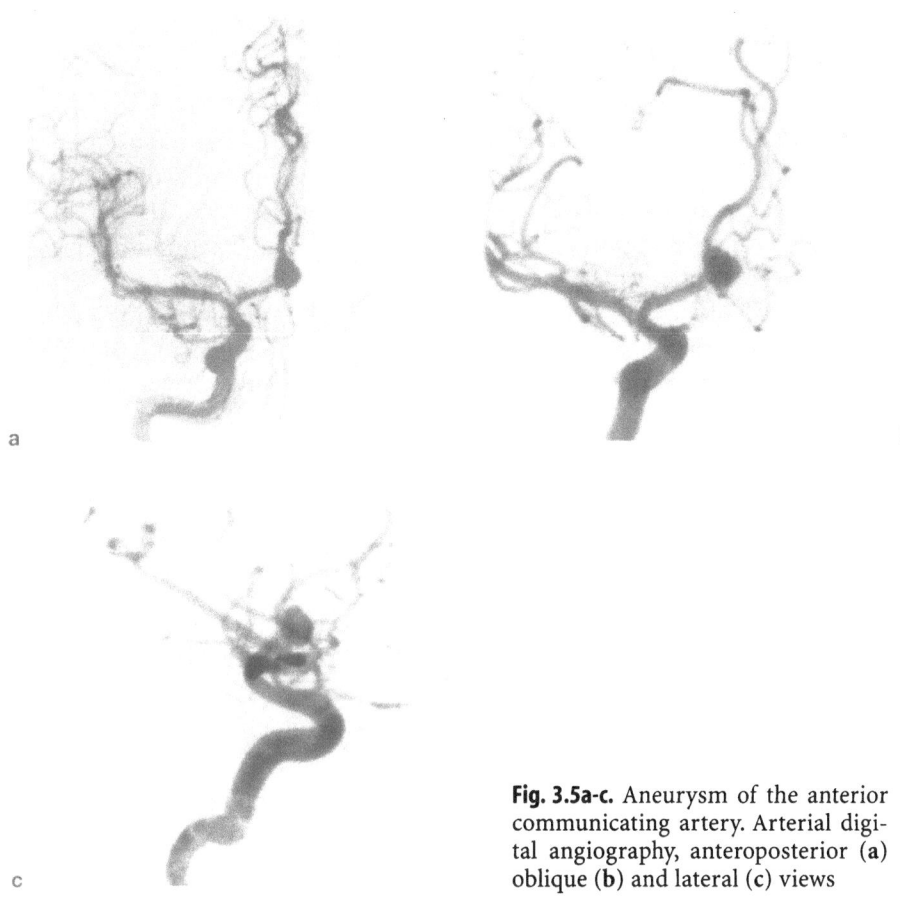

Fig. 3.5a-c. Aneurysm of the anterior communicating artery. Arterial digital angiography, anteroposterior (**a**) oblique (**b**) and lateral (**c**) views

apeutic strategy is the prompt surgical exclusion of the aneurysm from the arterial circle, if the patient is placed between zero and third grades of Hunt and Hess' scale. If the patient is in worse neurological conditions (grades IV-V), the surgical operation must be delayed to give the brain time and opportunity to recover after the hemorrhagic stress. The symptomatic vasospasm represents the main cause of failure in the treatment of SAH and, to date, there is no effective treatment for it. This is due to the fact that the mechanisms responsible for the spasm of the subarachnoid arterial vessels are still not completely known.

Although various vasoactive factors have been found in the cerebrospinal fluid of patients affected by SAH, in variable concentractions in relation to the time elapsed from the bleeding, no specific treatment has given encouraging results so far.

In the 1980s, calcium antagonists (nimodipine, nifedipine, nicardipine) were used for the treatment of the vasospasm post-SAH; their real effectiveness has not been carefully tested yet.

Nowadays, the best therapy still seems to be arterial hypertension and hypervolemia which, expanding the circulating hematic volume and increasing the intrarterial pressure, decrease the incidence of the cerebral ischemia and solve, more or less completely, the connected neurological disorders (70% of cases).

Neuroradiologists have recently adopted a technique of dilation of the arteries in spasm by using a balloon (transluminal angioplasty). This technique can have a therapeutic role when drugs do not give results.

Therapy

Therapy for anterial cerebral aneurysms aims to exclude the aneurysmatic sac from the blood circulation. This result can be achieved with surgical or endovascular treatment.

Surgical therapy

With the aid of a microscope, the neck of the aneurysmal sac can be closed with a metallic clip or ligature (Figs. 3.6-3.9). When the closure of the neck is not possible, we can strengthen the sac by wrapping it with foreign bodies, like cotton or acrylic substances, stimulating a hyperplastic inflammatory reaction of the aneurysmal wall with consequent decrease of bleeding risk. The results are excellent: 95%-97% of success in patients operated in good neurological conditions (grade I-II according to Hunt and Hess).

Endovascular treatment

This technique consists in reaching, after femoral artery catheterization, the vessel from which the aneurysm arises, then penetrating in the aneurysmal sac with a inflated microballons in order to fill the aneurysmal sac excluding it from the circle. Electrically charged platinum coils are used in alternative. These coils, after being placed in the aneurysm, provoke the formation of a thrombus which occludes the aneurysmal sac (Fig. 3.10a,b,c). The results achieved by the above techniques are similar to those achieved by surgical procedure.

Fig. 3.6. a Microsurgical appearance of the comunicating anterior artery. **b** Micro-surgical appearance after clipping (asterisks indicate aneurysms)

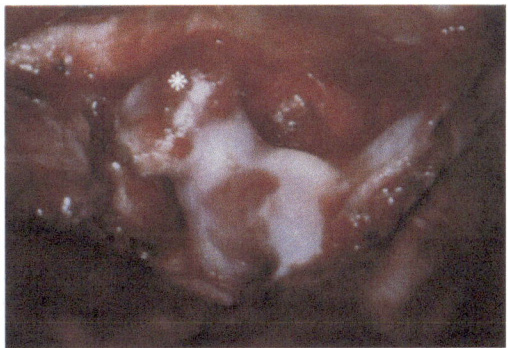

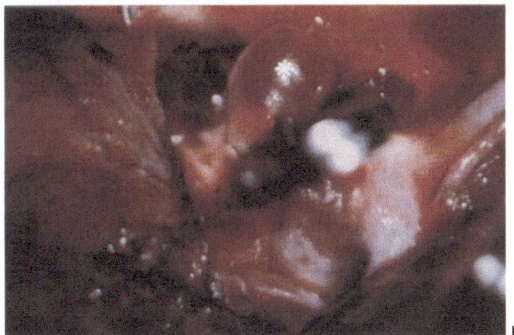

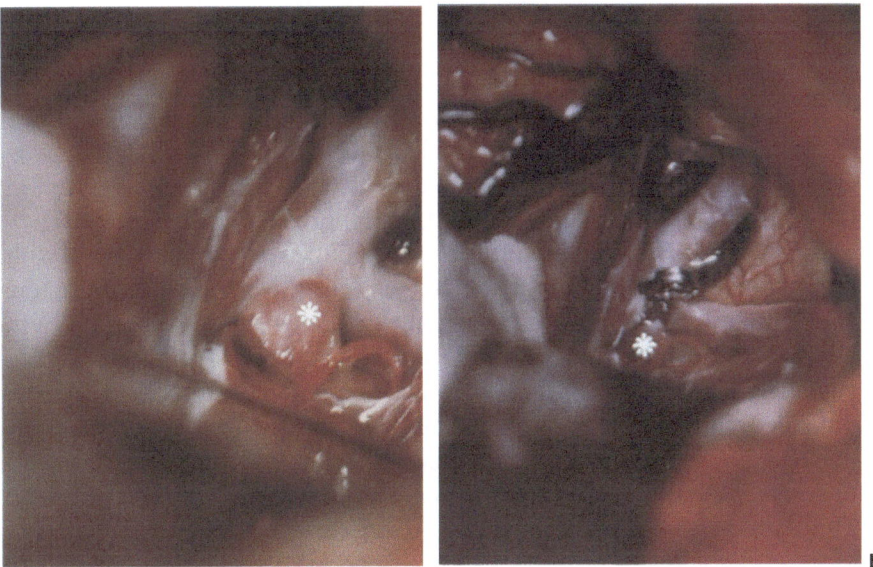

Fig. 3.7 a Microsurgical aspect of carotid bifurcation. **b** Microsurgical post-clipping appearance (asterisks indicate aneurysms)

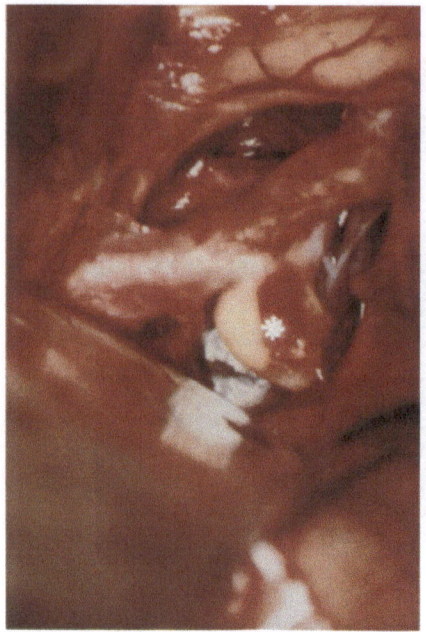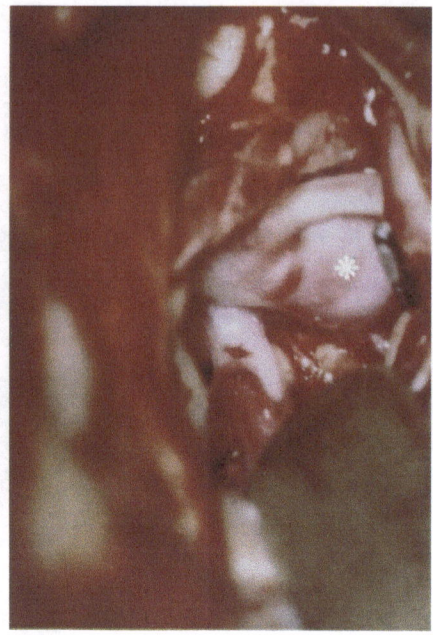

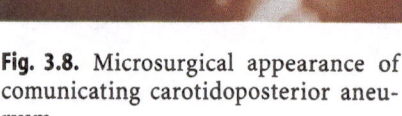

Fig. 3.8. Microsurgical appearance of comunicating carotidoposterior aneurysm

Fig. 3.9. Microsurgical appearance of a top basilar aneurysm

Aneurysms in pediatric age

In the largest surveys, a frequency of 0.5%-4.6%, a preference for males (male-female ratio is 3:1), a high incidence at the level of the posterior circle and a high percentage of aneurysms of the anterior circle localized in the bifurcation of the internal carotid, are reported.

Giant aneurysms represent 30%-45%, and they are associated with intraparenchymal or subdural hematomas. Vascular spasm is found, using angiography, in 10%-15% of cases only and, when it is present, it is not always followed by ischemic lesions. The etiopathogenesis of aneurysms in pediatric age is similar to that in adults, even if some authors suggested a possible traumatic etiology for posterior circle aneurysms. For example, during labor the intracranial hypertension could push the posterior cerebral artery against the tentorium free edge, damaging the vascular wall. This damage may cause, in time, the formation of aneurysms.

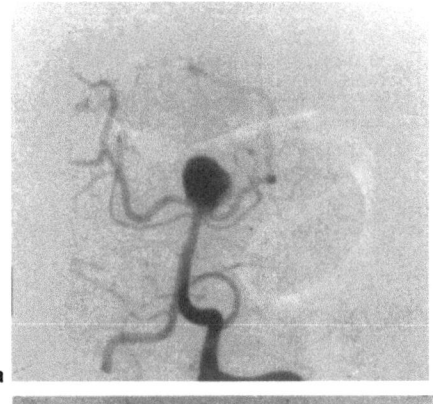
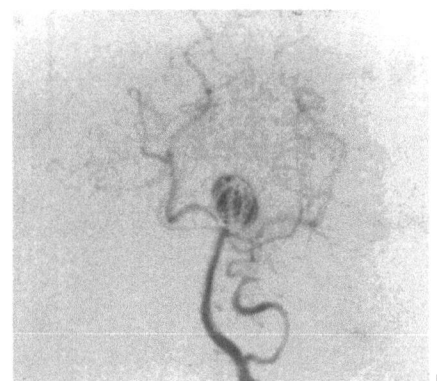
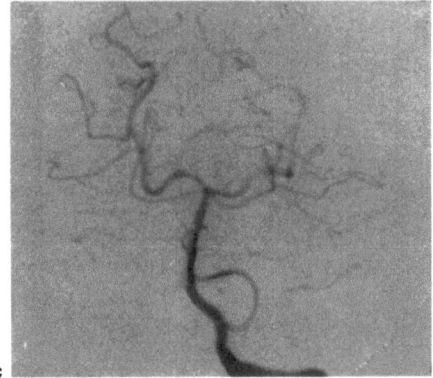

Fig. 3.10. Basilar top aneurysm. Arterial digital angiography. **a** Giant aneurysm of the basilar top. **b, c** Endovascular exclusion of the aneurysmatic sac with detached spirals. Intermediate phase (**b**); final phase (**c**)

Mycotic aneurysms

The mycotic aneurysms are much rarer than the previous ones: they account for 1%-2% of cases and represent a complication of infective endocarditis of rheumatic origin. They can also be the consequence of meningitis, cranial osteomyelitis, or a cavernous sinus infective syndrome. The pathogenesis is unknown. They can derive from a contiguous arteritis in case of meningitis or infections of the cavernous sinus. In case of endocarditis, they can derive from septic emboli which could involve the Vircow-Robin spaces causing an adventitial inflammation.

The mycotic aneurysms tend to form at the level of the peripheral branches of the major vessels. The surgical treatment is controversial: some authors advise a conservative treatment with antibiotic drugs but, in case this is not effective, a surgical operation is necessary. In case of an intracerebral hematoma with mass effect, it is advisable to proceed to an urgent operation in order to empty the hematoma and exclude the aneurysm.

4. Vascular malformations of the central nervous system

Epidemiology

Vascular malformations or "angiomas" of the central nervous system consist in a pathological tangle of arteries, veins, capillaries and/or canals of a presumably congenital nature. They are "dynamic" lesions, being characterized by a continuous change in diameter and appearance. The incidence of angiomas in Europe and North America is about 4000-5000 cases per year, one-tenth of the incidence of intracranial aneurysms.

The vascular malformations of the central nervous system are classified into four clinicopathological categories: arteriovenous malformations (AVM), cavernous angiomas, venous angiomas, and capillary angiomas or telangectasias. From a clinical point of view, the most frequent angiomas are the AVMs, but autopsical reports demonstrate that venous angiomas and telangectasias are the most frequent although they remain asymptomatic.

Arteriovenous malformations

AVMs consist in pathological vessels which form arteriovenous shunts without intermediate capillaries or nervous parenchyma. Number, length and diameter of vessels, usually forming a tangle, are very variable. Feeding vessels and draining veins are dilated and sinuous.

Histologically, the vasal component is of a transitional type. Sometimes the vasal wall is limited by connective tissue only; in other cases the elastic lining is hypotrophic, reduced in thickness or absent.

In relation to their size they are classified into: small-medium (diameter between 3 and 6 cm), and large (over 6 cm). They can localize everywhere in the brain, mainly in supratentorial regions (in territories vascularized by the middle and anterior cerebral arteries).

The majority of AVMs becomes symptomatic in subjects when they are 40 years of age. They do not show any preference in gender (contrary to aneurysms) and there is no familiar or genetic predisposition.

Symptomatology

The first AVM symptom is hemorrhage, followed by epilepsy, headache and local ischemic deficits.

Intraparenchymal hemorrhage due to rupture of the angioma is the most common symptom (30%-55% of cases at every age and 70% under 40 years of age). Subarachnoid and intraventricular hemorrhages are associated with intracerebral hematic collection. The risk of hemorrhage in patients affected by AVM is 1%-3% every year and the risk of rebleeding is 6%. Annually, the mortality and morbility incidence, for untreated AVMs, is 1% and 2%-3%, respectively. Small AVMs bleed more than the voluminous ones. The hemorrhage is often associated with physical or psychic stress or pregnancy.

The clinical picture is acute and is characterized by headache and sometimes loss of consciousness. Sensorimotor deficits, visual field deficits, motor and/or sensory aphasia, and cranial nerve or cerebellar deficits occur in relation to the hemorrhage's localization.

Partial or generalized epilepsy is the second symptom (25%-50% of cases), especially if the AVM is localized in the temporal, frontal or parietal lobes.

In most cases epilepsy is sensitive to drug therapy, but sometimes surgical treatment is necessary for a definitive recovery. Headache is a frequent symptom in patients affected by AVM (10%-20% of cases). Headache is often in the form of hemicrania (mainly in occipital lobe AVMs), is unilateral, and is associated with precritical aura or visual disturbances.

In about 10% of cases, there are focal deficits due to ischemia. They are caused by hypoperfusion of the parenchyma surrounding the lesion due to blood withdrawal by the high-flow AVMs.

Communicating or non-communicating hydrocephalus and related symptoms are present in 10% of cases.

Radiological diagnosis

Cerebral angiography is the best test to define and to plan the therapy of a cerebral AVM. CT and NMR are utilized as screening tests for the diagnosis. At CT, the malformation with a recent bleeding appears like a hematoma(hyperdense and with mass effect). Angioma appears as an

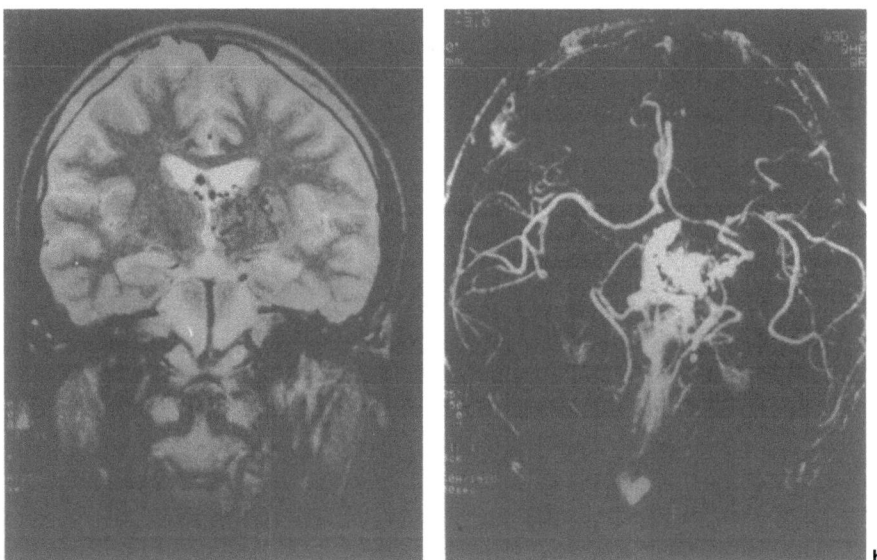

a   b

Fig. 4.1a,b. Cerebral AVM. MRI, T2-weighted image, coronal view (**a**), and angio-MRI, axial view (**b**). Presence of arteriovenous malformation at basal nuclei

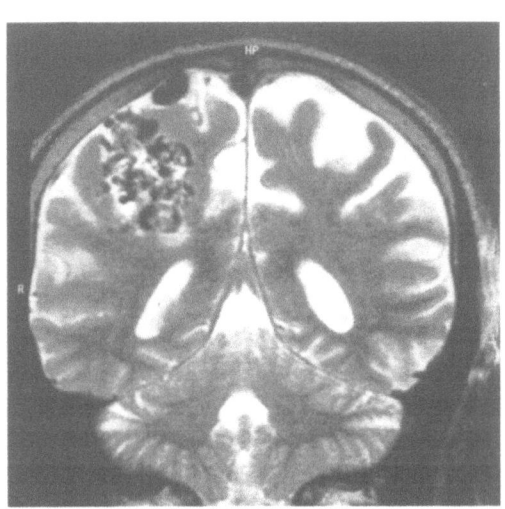

Fig. 4.2. Right rolandic arteriovenous malformation. MRI, T2-weighted image. Multiple areas of signal void and with serpiginous morphology, expression of ectatic vascular structures

irregular, hypo- or hyperdense area in the brain tissue which presents contrast enhancement. Hyperdense, serpiginous images sometimes appear, indicating the presence of pathological vessels.

NMR provides a clear, three-dimensional image of the location and components of the AVM such as feeding arteries, draining veins and nidus. If there is a hemorrhage, NMR shows hypointense areas inside the lesion or in surrounding structures. The hypointense signal on T2-weighted images is due to accumulated hemosiderin (Figs. 4.1; 4.2).

Angio-NMR and cerebral angiography allow a precise diagnosis, showing the nidus, the feeding and draining vessels, satellite aneurysms and other associated malformations (Figs. 4.3; 4.4).

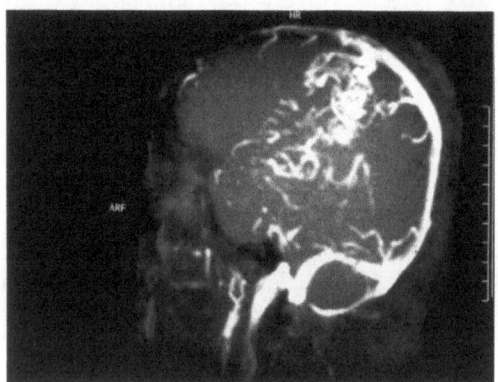

Fig. 4.3. Right rolandic arteriovenous malformation. Angio-MRI confirms the presence of ectatic vascular structures, localized in right rolandic site with venous drain in the superior longitudinal sinus

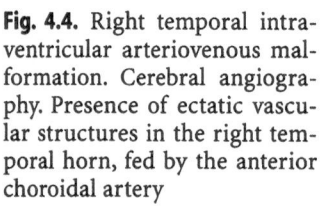

Fig. 4.4. Right temporal intraventricular arteriovenous malformation. Cerebral angiography. Presence of ectatic vascular structures in the right temporal horn, fed by the anterior choroidal artery

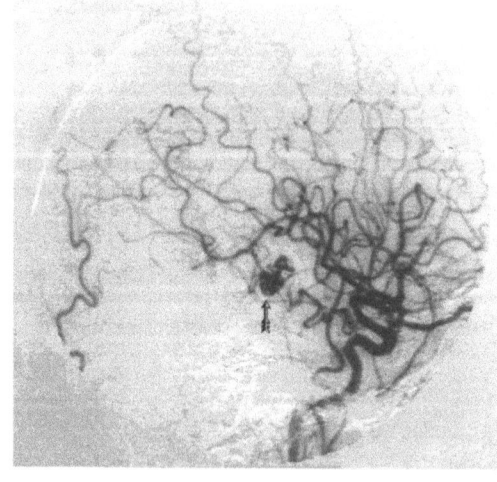

Therapy

The neurosurgeon must estimate the risks connected to the treatment of choice and the natural history of the malformation. The therapeutic alternatives include: 1) surgical treatment, 2) embolization, and 3) radio-surgery.

Surgical treatment

Surgery is the only definitive treatment (Fig. 4.5), but it can be associated with morbidity or mortality. The selective criteria for a surgical treatment are: a) clinical history and first symptoms, b) age, c) localization of the AVM, and d) size and shape of the AVM.

a) *Clinical history and first symptoms.* If the first symptom is hemorrage, the risk of rebleeding is higher compared to cases in which the first symptom is epilepsy or headache. Nevertheless, this rule is not always confirmed.

b) *Age.* Surgical treatment is more necessary in young patients. It is not advisable to operate on asymptomatic patients of 55-60 years of age. In

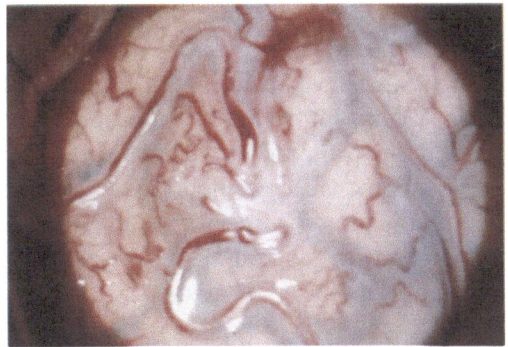
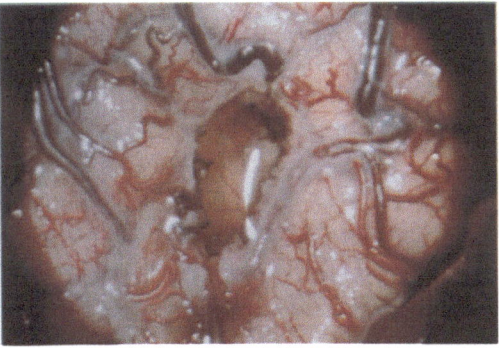

Fig. 4.5a,b. Microsurgical aspect of a cortical cerebral angioma, before (**a**) and after (**b**) removal

fact, the surgical risk at age 55 is similar to that of the natural history of an unoperated AVM.

c) *Location.* When an AVM is located in an unapprochable site (basal nuclei, brainstem), the risk of postoperative neurological deficits is high. Therefore, AVMs should be operated only in young patients with hemorrhage as a first symptom, and by an expert neurosurgical team. Small lesions, located in silent cerebral areas, can also be operated in patients of advanced age.

d) *Size and shape.* Large angiomas, with a high number of feeding arteries, deep draining veins and several nidi, imply many surgical difficulties and a high risk of postoperative neurological deficits.

Endovascular embolization

Endovascular embolization rarely leads to the complete obliteration of the AVM. Recanalization can occur, forming new arteriovenous shunts after vessel occlusion. Therefore, embolization cannot be the only treatment of middle and large AVMs, but it can be an important adjuvant to the preoperative therapy. The embolization can be performed with superselective transfemoral cerebral angiography using embolic and not reabsorbable agents (such as silicone), microballoons or platinum coils.

Radiosurgery

It is an alternative treatment for cerebral angiomas. In stereotactic radiosurgery, high energy radiation (produced by a gamma-knife and formed by protonic rays) is directed on the nidus of the angioma. Radiosurgery causes gradual vessel sclerosis which, after 1-2 years, leads to obliteration. Radiosurgery can be performed in patients affected by small angiomas with general surgical risks (systemic diseases, advanced age) and/or local risks (critical areas).

Cavernous angiomas or cavernomas

They are single or multiple vascular malformations. Usually, they are small and appear as circumscribed nodules (blackberry-like) they do not have a capsule and are reddish in color.

Microscopically, they consist in sinusoidal vascular lakes without intercalated cerebral tissue. The sinusoidal component has no elastic or muscular layer and is delimited by an endothelial layer. The size varies from a pin head to a mass with a diameter of some centimeters. The incidence is about 0.02%-0.04%.

The most affected age is the third-fourth decade of life and there is no preference of gender. They are multiple in 17% of cases and familiarity is present in 12% of cases. Cavernous angioma can localize in every area of the central and peripheral nervous system. In 75% of cases, they are localized in supratentorial areas (cortical and subcortical regions of temporal, frontal, parietal, occipital lobes, rarely at the basal nuclei). In 25% of cases, they localize in subtentorial areas (brainstem, cerebellum).

Symptomatology

Cavernous angiomas can be asymptomatic and accidentally diagnosed with cerebral CT or NMR.

Symptomatology is variable; the first symptom is usually epilepsy, followed by headache and hemorrhage. The epileptic seizure varies in relation to the location. Cavernous angiomas localized in the temporal lobe cause partial seizures. Cavernous angiomas localized in the frontal lobe cause generalized seizures and sensorimotor seizures, if localized in the rolandic region.

Headache can be gravative or hemicranic. Hemorrhage usually is intraparenchymal and small; rarely it is subarachnoid.

Symptomatology is dependent on the location of the hemorrhage.

Radiological diagnosis

Usually, angiography does not show any cavernous angioma and it is negative in 80%-90% of cases. This is due to the absence of direct arterial afferences and their slow flow. In 10%-20% of cases, angiography is positive and shows: a) capillary blush in late phase; b) early venous drainage; and c) sometimes a small arterial afferent vessel. CT and NMR, in the last 10 years, have increased the diagnostic potential.

CT shows cavernous angioma as circumscribed areas, sometimes dyshomogeneous, with hypo- or hyperdense zones with contrast enhancement.

At NMR, the cavernomas appearance is peculiar, particularly on T2-weighted images. NMR shows a variegated, hypo- or hyperintense mass which is, generally, surrounded by a peripheric hypointensity. This hypointensity is due to hemosiderin accumulation (Figs. 4.6; 4.7a,b).

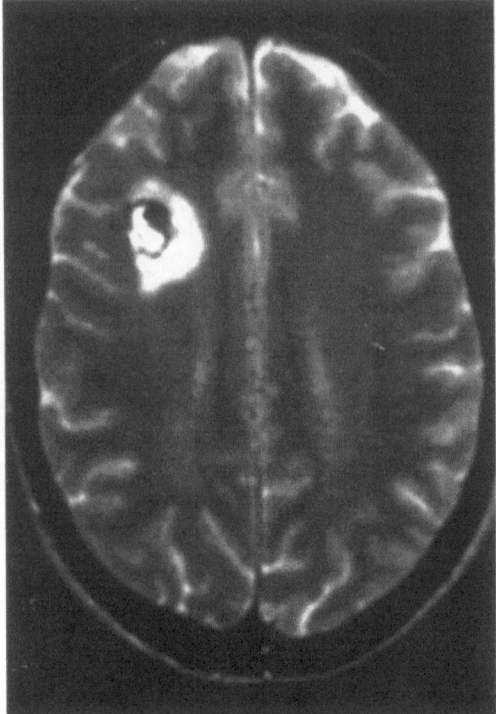

Fig. 4.6. Cavernoma. NMR, T2-weighted image. Right frontal area of dyshomogeneous intensity due to the presence of hemoglobin bioproducts, at different stages of degradation. Surrounding edema is present

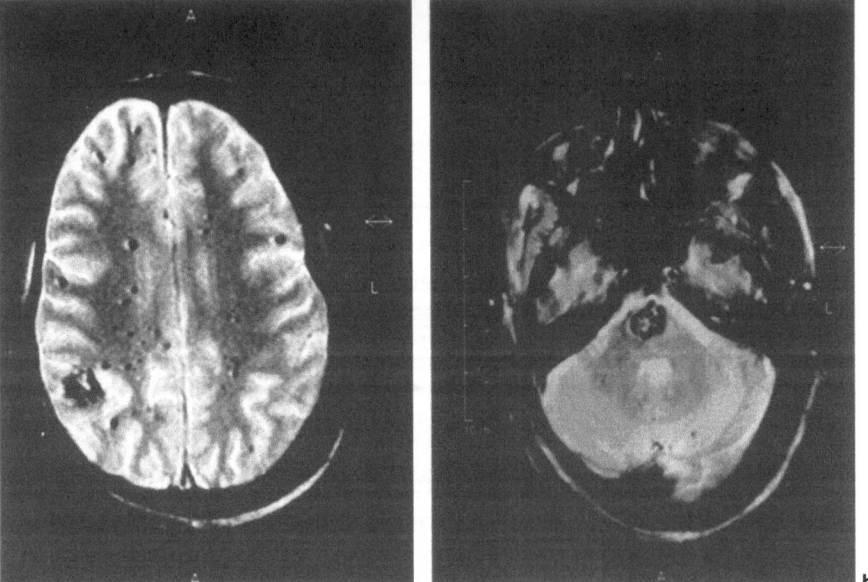

a   b

Fig. 4.7a,b. Multiple cavernomas. MRI, T2-weighted images. Presence of multiple, hypointense areas in cerebral hemispheres (**a**) and a voluminose area in the pons (**b**)

Therapy

The treatment of cavernomas depends on symptomatology and location. Hemorrhagic cavernomas need to be removed with surgical treatment.

Cavernomas which cause drug-resistent epilepsy also require surgical treatment. Treatment is conservative and associated with periodical check-ups in case of cavernomas which cause epilepsy sensitive to drug therapy or that are localized in critical areas.

Venous angiomas

They are the most frequent vascular malformations. They consist in anom-alous vessels surrounded by normal brain tissue. They can be formed by a single, tortuous and very dilated vein or by several small confluent venous vessels ("radial arrangement"). There never is a clear arterial afference.

Histologically, the venous component consists in a smooth muscle wall and elastic tissue. Venous angioma is asymptomatic; however, seizures and hemorrhage can occur.

Radiological diagnosis

Angiography shows a typical image called "caput medusae". The lesion appears as several radial veins which converge in a draining vein localized centrally or in a dural sinus.

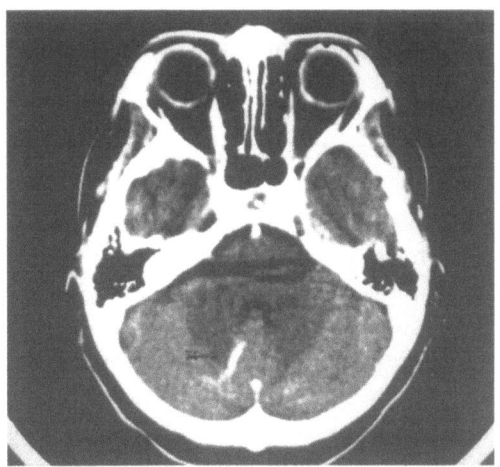

Fig. 4.8. Venose angioma. CT after contrast medium shows a right paravermiana venous ectasia with peripheral aspect similar to the caput medusae

CT shows a transparenchymal venous trunk ("white-line sign") (Fig. 4.8). NMR shows a linear venous trunk in the white matter, as a hypo-intense line or a signal void ("black-line sign").

Therapy

Treatment is conservative except in case of several hemorrhages or drug-resistant epilepsy.

Capillary angiomas or telangectasias

They are very small vascular malformations (generally smaller than 1 cm in diameter). They are often multiple and formed by small capillary vessels.

Histologically, the vessels are similar to normal capillaries and there is normal brain tissue among them. Sometimes, telangectasias are associated with other vascular malformations such as cavernomas. They are often localized in the pons and periventricular white matter. Telangectasias usually are asymptomatic and rarely cause hemorrhage or thrombosis; their observation is often autopsical.

Radiological diagnosis

Usually angiography does not clearly show capillary angioma (cryptic angiomas). CT, after contrast medium administration, and NMR show telangectasias as hyperdense and hypointense (signal void) vascular signals, respectively, but they are rarely observed.

Dural arteriovenous malformations

They are vascular malformations due to a direct communication between the arterial and the venous systems at the level of the dura mater. They can be classified in relation to the involved venous sinuses: sigmoid and transverse, superior sagittal, and cavernous sinuses.

The etiopathogenic factors responsible for this anomalous communication can be either congenital, in relation to anomalies of the venous draining system, or aquired. Among the latter, we can list cranial traumas or inflammatory and thrombotic processes at the level of the venous sinus, with its partial or total closure and consequent opening of small arteriovenous fistulas, already present in the venous sinus.

The symptomatology varies in relation to the venous sinus involved. A common characteristic is cerebral hemorrhage (subarachnoid, subdural, or intraparenchymal), headache and perception of a cranial sound. In the dural fistulas affecting the cavernous sinus, we can observe head pain localized principally at the level of the orbital cavity, conjunctival chemosis, light exophthalmos and deficit in cranial nerve VI. In the dural fistulas affecting the sigmoid and transverse sinuses, the initial symptom can be headache or occipital sound and symptoms of intracranial hypertension.

In the petrous, sphenoparietal and superior sagittal sinuses, the initial symptom is a tiresome sound. Sometimes, however, they can be asymptomatic, until the appearance of hemorrhage.

A definite diagnosis of dural AVM is based on angiography which allows the identification of the arterial shunt in the venous sinus, the retrograde flow across the pial veins and the irregularities or closure of the venous sinus. A tentative diagnosis can be obtained with cerebral CT or cerebral NMR. The therapy is surgical and consists in the closure of the arterial afferences either directly or by an endovascular approach with embolization.

Aneurysm of Galen's vein

The aneurysm of Galen's vein can be considered to be an aneurysmatic dilation of Galen's vein which receives arterial supply from one or more of the greater intracranial arteries, directly or through the interposition of an angiomatous malformation.

The clinical picture is characterized by cardiac insufficiency, hydrocephalus, intracranial hemorrhage, phenomena caused by blood withdrawal and local compression. The clinical picture varies according to the patient's age at the time when the aneurysm occurs.

During the neonatal period, the clinical picture is characterized by high output heart failure. A strong continuous murmur can be auscultated on the whole skull. During the first two years of life, the clinical picture is characterized by macrocephaly, secondary to hydrocephalus.

During childhood, after two years of age, the aneurysm can occur with subarachnoid hemorrhage or craniomegaly; a constant murmur, can be perceived on the skull.

In older children and in young adults, the clinical picture can consist in subarachnoid hemorrhage, hydrocephalus and signs of compression in the pineal region.

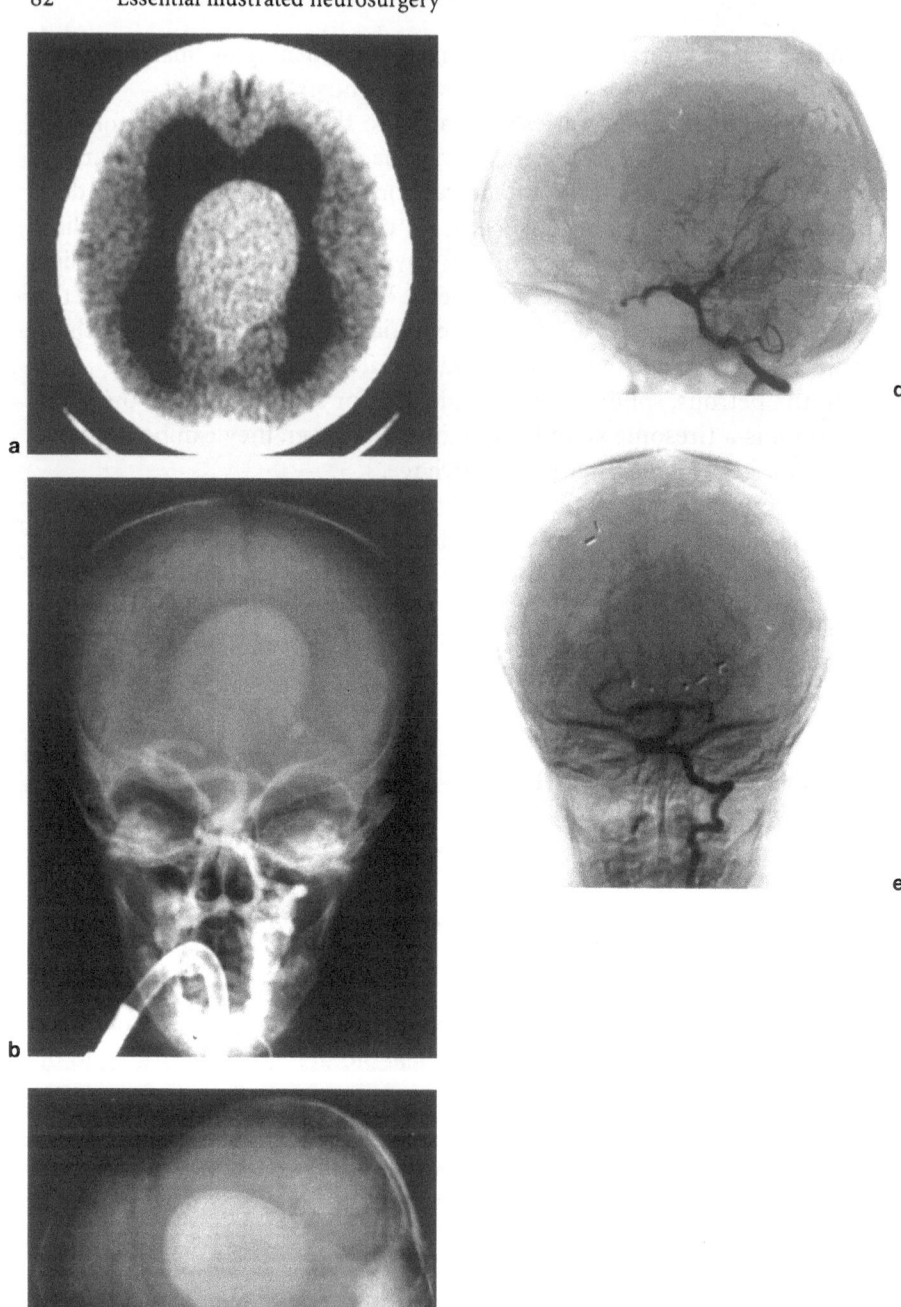

Fig. 4.9a-e. Aneurysm of the ampulla of Galen. CT without contrast medium (**a**). Cerebral angiography before (**b**, **c**) and after surgical treatment (**d**, **e**)

The diagnosis, apart from the clinical aspects, is based on CT (Fig. 4.9a), angiography (Fig. 4.9b,c) and cerebral angio-NMR, which show the aneurysm, the afferences and the venous drains.

"Moya-moya" disease

This disease is caused by a dysplasia of both internal carotid arteries associated with stenosis or obliteration. It was described for the first time in 1955 and, for 10 years, it was believed to affect Japanese people only. The word "moya-moya", coined by Suzuki in 1969, describes the angiographic appearance of the malformation, resembling a cloud of smoke. Since 1965, clinical studies have reported the presence of this disease in America and Europe as well, but less frequently than in Japan. Stenosis can also be found in renal or coronary arteries. Recently, it has been demons trated that this lesion can involve the external carotid artery as well. This suggests that the molecular mechanism which causes thickening of the intima of the intracranial arteries also involves the extracranial carotid circle. The amount of fibroblast growth factor (bFGF) is increased in the superficial temporal artery of patients affected by this disease. bFGF stimulates mitosis in many cell types and can regulate smooth muscle and endothelial cell proliferation and migration. An increase in bFGF production is believed to be responsible for the thickening of the intima of the arteries. It seems that the presence of the copious nervous fibers surrounding the internal carotid bifurcation can explain the more frequent involvement of the intracranial circle by vascular stenosis. These fibers contain neurotransmitters, such as substance P, which have a mitogenic activity on the vascular smooth muscle cells. This disease has two incidence peaks: in subjects under 10 years and in those around 30 years of age; it is more frequent in women. Clinically, moya-moya disease can appear with transient ischemic attacks, cerebral stroke, seizures or hemorrhage. The first three manifestations are frequent in children while the fourth is frequent in adults.

The angiographic picture shows stenosis or obliteration of the internal carotid supraclinoid tract, with frequent involvement of the anterior and middle cerebral arteries. An abnormal cloud of vascular formations is present in the basal cranium. These are fed by choroidal, lenticulostriate and thalamostriate arteries (Fig. 4.10a,b).

The radiological aspect is not uniform because the disease can be diagnosed in one of six developmental phases. For example, in the sixth and last stage there is no typical aspect as described above, and the circulation is ensured only by leptomeningeal anastomosis. CT can evidence multiple

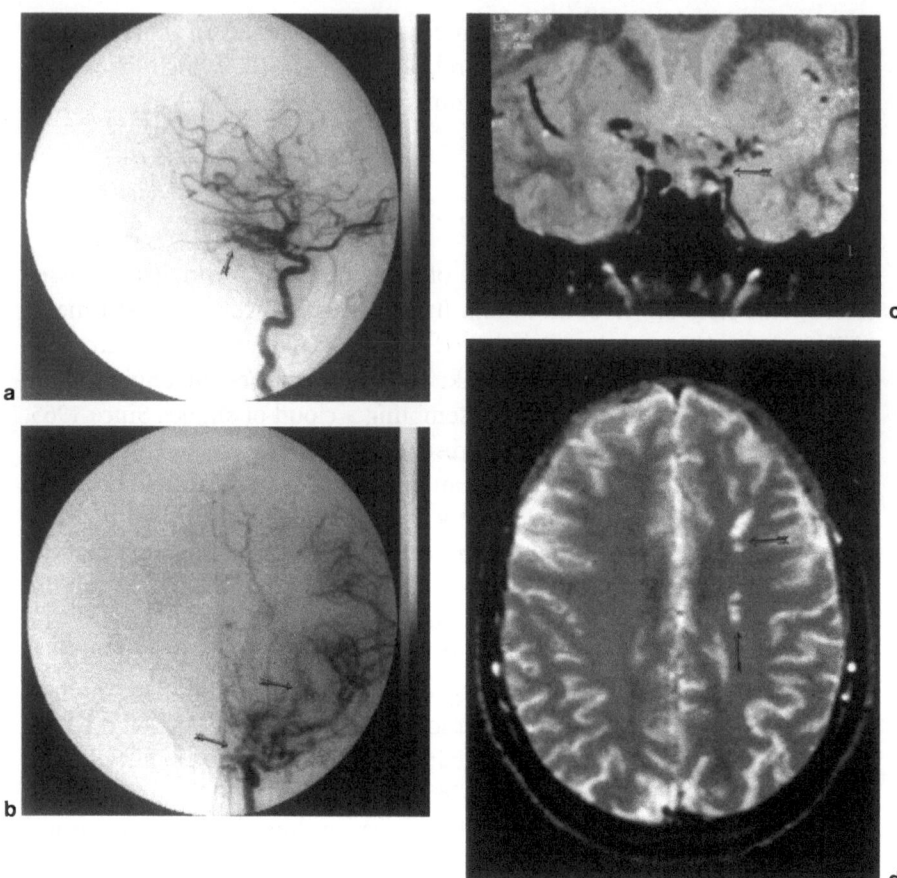

Fig. 4.10a-d. Moya-moya disease. Cerebral angiography (**a-b**): the distal tract of the left carotid siphon is dyshomogeneous and there are various hypertrophic collateral branches. Marked hypertrophy of perforating lenticulostriate branches. MRI, coronal (**c**) and axial (**d**) views, T2-weighted images. Incomplete visualization of the supraclinoid tract of the left intenal carotid artery (**c**) and presence of multiple lacunar ischemic lesions in the white matterof the left radiate crown (**d**)

hypodense leptomeningeal areas and cerebral atrophy with secondary ventricular dilation.

NMR can show the complete visualization or the absence of vascular signal in the carotid siphon and presence of hypertrophic collateral branches, mainly in the lenticulostriate artery territory (Fig. 4.10c). Ischemic lacunar lesions can appear in the white matter of the involved cerebral hemisphere (Fig. 4.10d). In a later phase, cerebral atrophy can be observed.

The natural evolution of the disease is variable: some patients have no sequelae (19%), while others have transient ischemic attacks (33%) or dementia which requires continuous parental care. Death occurs in 3% of cases. The surgical treatment can be various: anastomosis between superficial temporal artery and middle cerebral artery (STA-MCA), encephalomyosinangiosis (the temporal muscle is overturned on the cerebral surface) or encephalogaleosynangiosis (the temporal artery is overturned with the galea on the brain surface), or omentum graft. The aim of all these treatments is to ensure a compensation in order to recover the neurological deficits and prevent transient ischemic attacks. It is difficult to establish which is the best procedure. The best treatment is probably a combination of direct and indirect revascularization procedures.

5. Craniosynostosis

Etiopathogenesis

In 1791, Virchow was the first to suppose that the premature synostosis of a cranial suture limited the perpendicular growth at the level of that suture and it caused, instead, an excessive growth in the direction of the suture itself. He also concluded that the premature closure of the suture was the consequence of a local inflammatory process.

The etiology of the premature closure of a suture is still unknown. Most of the sutures form during the tenth to sixteenth weeks of fetal life and the dura mater represents the guidance tissue for the morphogenesis of the skull. Moss supports the idea that there is no genetic determination of dimensions, shapes and osseous growth and that macro- and microcephaly are the consequence of hyper- or hypovolumetric growth of the cerebral mass. The dura mater is tenaciously connected to the cranial basis in five points: the apophysis of the crista galli, the sphenoidal wings and the cristae of the petrous bone. The dural fibers departing from these points will then control the skull growth and will ossify very slowly because of the mechanical stress to which they are subjected. Consequently, this means that the sutures are not necessarily the first cause of the cranyosinostosis etiology, since they passively respond to normal or abnormal mechanical forces. Whatever the cause is, the premature closure of a suture has two main effects: 1) it inhibits the further expansion perpendicularly to the suture and 2) it changes the direction of growth of the cerebral mass.

Children affected by craniosynostosis are usually examined by the neurosurgeon because parents are warried about the craniofacial deformities and possibilities of disabling sequelae such as epilepsy, mental retardation, visual disorders and endocranial hypertension.

The simple inspection of the patient's head in all directions is sufficient to diagnose a morphological deformity of the skull. In children under 3 months of age, the absence of mobility of the cranial bones at palpation and the finding of a small osseous crista in correspondence of a suture, especially the sagittal one, are strongly indicative of craniosynostosis. On the contrary, the presence of a small or not palpable fontanel, even in a newborn, has no diagnostic value.

The radiograms of the skull are important for the diagnosis of craniosynostosis diagnosis. However, they should be done three weeks after birth, when the cranial bone is more radiodense, since there are seldom indications for surgical operation before this time. The radiological test must be done according to the standard projections and it must evidence the skull shape and the suture of the cranial convexity. A closed suture often appears as a hyperdense band. Cerebral CT gives, instead, useful information on the orbital and sphenoidal wing regions and, above all, it evidences a possible associated hydrocephalus or other malformations (Figs. 5.1, 5.2).

The indications for a surgical operation are only two: the cosmetic abnormalities and the intracranial hypertension associated with hydrocephalus.

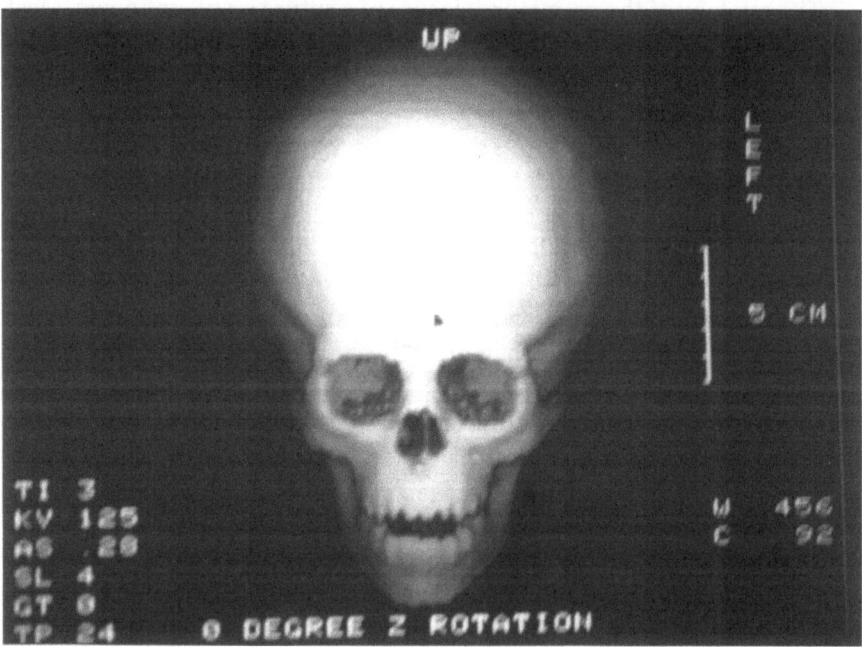

Fig. 5.1. Craniostenosis. Three-dimensional reconstruction. Turri-cephaly

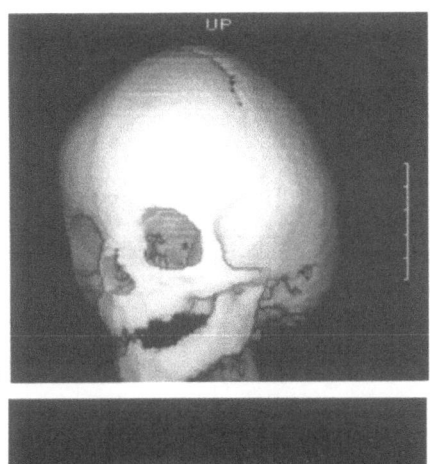

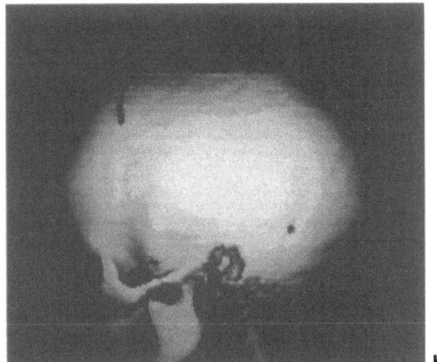

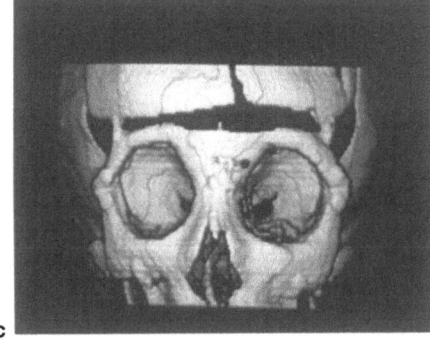

Fig. 5.2a-c. Craniostosis. CT, three-dimensional preoperative (**a, b**) and postoperative (**c**) reconstructions. Scaphocephaly (**a**). Outcome of craniectomy (**c**)

If craniosynostosis is not surgically treated, the deformities often worsen and cause a progressive distortion of the calvaria and the near stuctures like the orbits, skull and maxillary bones. The surgical correction of the anomaly by osteotomy and mobilization of the bone should be done after the third or fourth month of life, when the cranial expansion is more rapid and when the hematic volume is sufficient to compensate for the hematic loss during the operation.

Classification

Scaphocephaly

This deformity is due to precocious fusion of the sagittal suture with consequent cranial growth in anteroposterior directions (Figs. 5.3, 5.4). Upon cranial palpation, a bony crest is often found on the midline. The best cosmetic results can be obtained if the craniectomy, along the sagittal suture, is extended for at least 6-8 cm and if the parietal bone is mobilized bilaterally.

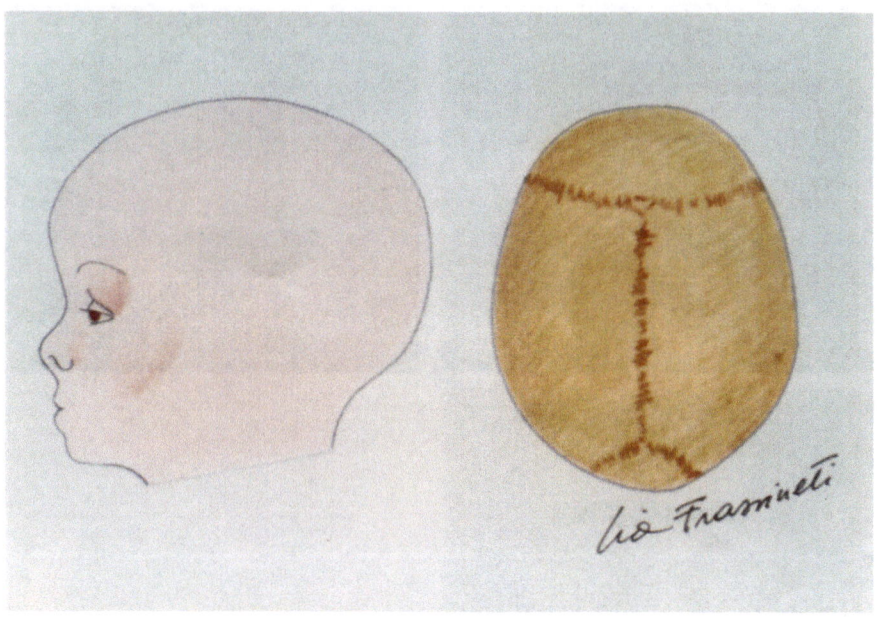

Fig. 5.3. Normal anatomical conformation of the skull

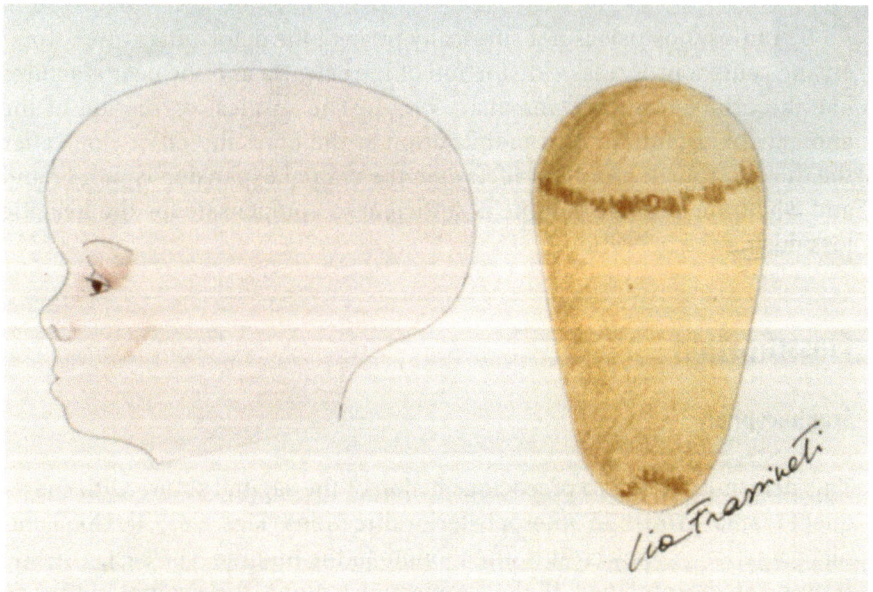

Fig. 5.4. Scaphocephaly

Brachycephaly, turricephaly and oxycephaly

They are morphological deformities associated with precocious and bilateral closure of the coronal suture. These words are sometimes used as synonyms, but sometimes they are considered to be totally separate entities. In the anteroposterior dimension the skull is narrow, while in the bitemporal dimension it is broader. The external occipital protuberance can be decreased or absent (Fig. 5.5). There can be a more or less serious involvement of the orbital arches and of the maxillary bones. The anterior fontanel is usually closed, while the bregmatic one can be exceptionally broad.

Palpation can reveal the presence of an osseous edge along the coronal suture, while the superior orbital arch, pushed backward, can cause facial deformities. Other sutures are very often jointed as well, causing intracranial hypertension.

The surgical operation aims to mobilize the frontal bone and the superior orbital margins as far as the frontozygomatic suture. After removing the convexity of the frontal bone, the frontal lobe must be lifted to expose both orbital roofs: osteotomy of the two superior arches must be performed from the frontonasal suture to the frontozygomatic suture.

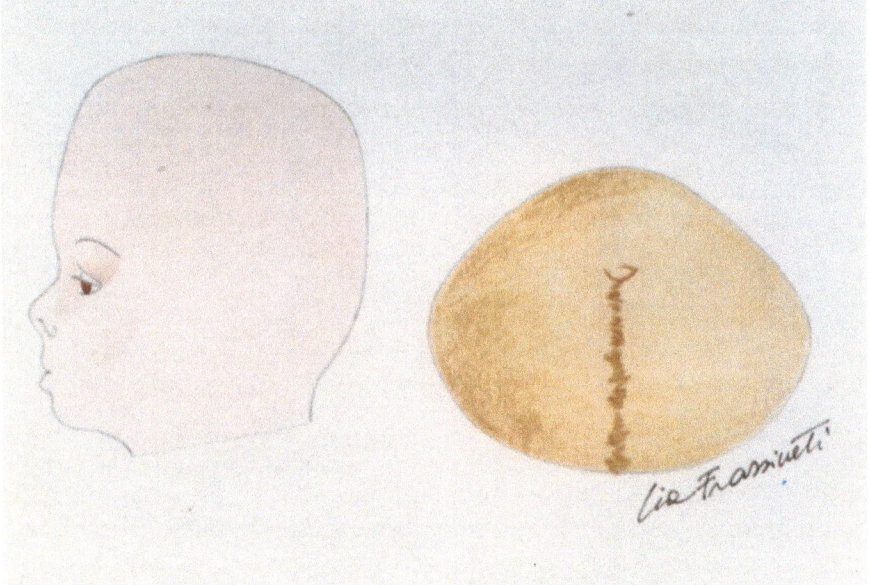

Fig. 5.5. Brachycephaly

Trigonocephaly

This malformation is associated with the premature closure of the metopic suture; if observed from the superior part, the skull is cuneiform, since the frontal region is narrower than usual, while the parietal region is broader (Fig. 5.6). There can be two kinds of trigonocephaly. The first kind, associated with anomalies of the frontal bone and of the orbits, is the most common. The second, instead, is characterized by a decreased development of the frontal lobes and it is associated with mental retardation.

Plagiocephaly

Anterior plagiocephaly

This anomaly is associated with the monolateral synostosis of the coronal suture, causeing cranial and facial asymmetry which, if not treated, can worsen during the child's growth (Fig. 5.7). At inspection, the involved frontal bone can appear flattened with a revolved orbit which is higher compared to the other, while the frontal contralateral bone and the parieto-occipital homolateral regions are swollen. Half of the children have a verti-

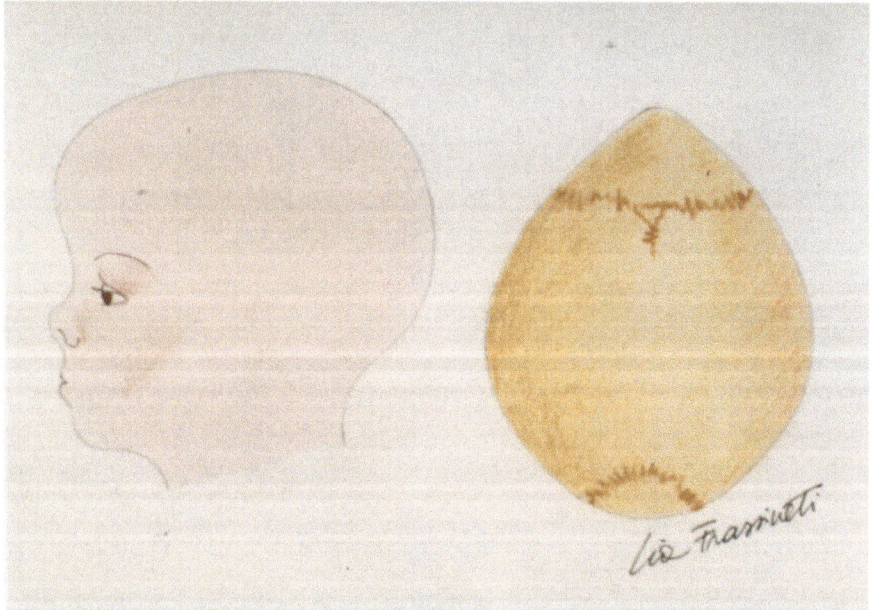

Fig. 5.6. Trigonocephaly

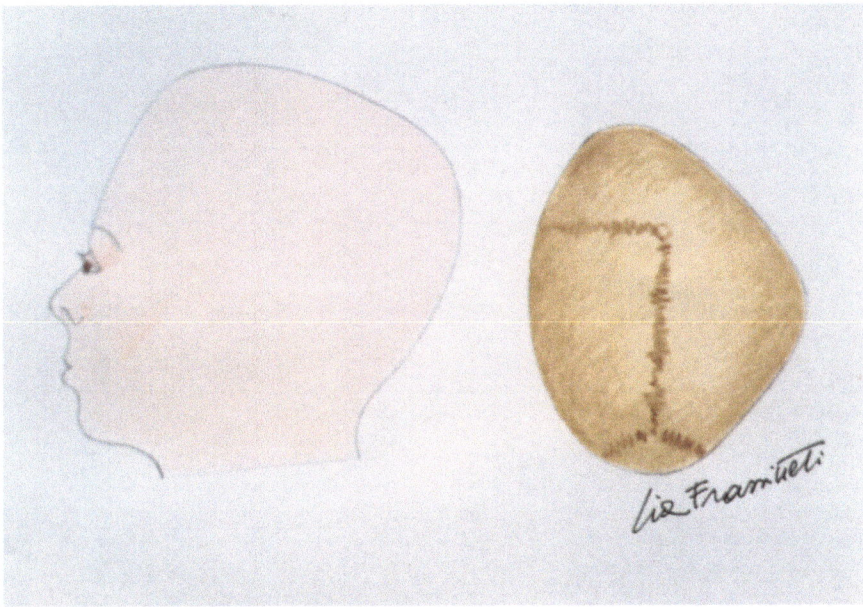

Fig. 5.7. Plagiocephaly

cal strabismus linked to the alteration of the orbital structure. The best results are obtained with an extensive operation of subperiost dissection, advancing of the orbit and reshaping the frontal bone. Some authors advise the removal of the lesser wing of the sphenoid bone and the orbital roof.

Posterior plagiocephaly

It is associated with the early closure of the lambdoid suture. It is rarer than the previous one, also due to the fact that this anomaly is exceptionally treated by the neurosurgeon being the esthetic defect covered by hair. We can adopt a conservative treatment if the plagiocephaly is precociously diagnosed, avoiding, for example, that the young patient leans on the flattened part of the skull while sleeping. Otherwise, the surgical operation must aim at surgical correction of the parietal and occipital bone asymmetry.

6. Hydrocephalus

Etiopathogenesis

Hydrocephalus is an abnormal and pressurized accumulation of cerebrospinal fluid inside the skull, with dilation of the ventricular cavities due to an alteration of cerebrospinal fluid dynamics. Any process which causes a discrepancy between the production and resorption of the cerebrospinal fluid leads to hydrocephalus. Usually, hydrocephalus derives from the obstruction of the cerebrospinal pathways; when the obstruction is inside the ventricular cavities, the hydrocephalus is called *"non-communicating"*; when the obstruction is at the level of the subarachnoid spaces, the hydrocephalus is called *"communicating"*.

The quantity of cerebrospinal fluid produced in one hour is about 20 ml, both in adults and in children. About 80%-90% of the cerebrospinal fluid is produced by the choroid plexi with an ultrafiltration process through the capillary wall. The remaining part is probably produced by the capillary endothelium of the cerebral parenchyma. The resorption of cerebrospinal fluid occurs, probably, by mechanisms of pressure gradients at the level of the villi and of the arachnoid granulations.

In relation to the mechanisms causing the abnormal accumulation of cerebrospinal fluid in the ventricular system, we can distinguish three types of hydrocephalus: *hypersecreting,* caused by excessive production of cerebrospinal fluid; *aresorptive,* caused by insufficient resorption of cerebrospinal fluid; and *obstructive,* caused by partial or total obstruction of the cerebrospinal pathways.

The *hypersecreting* hydrocephalus is rare. The pathological conditions which can cause it are mainly choroid plexi papillomas and intraventricular ependymomas.

The *aresorptive* hydrocephalus is also rare and is due to insufficient activity of the choroid plexi of the calvaria, which are responsible for cerebrospinal fluid resorption. The causes can be: the congenital absence of villi, an adhesive leptomeningitis wraping the villi, or the presence of erythrocytes and albumine in the cerebrospinal fluid, after a subarachnoid hemorrhage, blocking the function of the villi.

The *obstructive hydrocephalus* is due to a difficult cerebrospinal fluid flow caused by an obstacle localized at any point along the flow pathways: for example, at the level of one of Monro's foramen (*monoventricular hydrocephalus)* or at the level of both Monro's foramina or of the third ventricle (*biventricular hydrocephalus*). The biventrycular hydrocephalus is the caused by tumors such as colloid cysts, gliomas or tumors of the lateral ventricles or of the third ventricle (e.g. giant adenomas, craniopharyngiomas, tumors of the optic nerves, giant aneurysms of the anterior communicating artery) or residual scarring from inflammatory processes of the ependyma. The *triventricular hydrocephalus* is determined at the level of the sylvian aqueduct by stricture or congenital atresia of the aqueduct, cicatricial stenosis secondary to inflammatory processes of the ependyma, periaqueductal gliosis, or expansive processes in the posterior cranial fossa of tumoral or aneurysmatic nature (e.g. tumors of the fourth ventricle, of the pontocerebral angle, of the brainstem, aneurysms of the vertebro-basilar circle). At the level of Luska's and Magendi's foramina (*tetraventricular hydrocephalus*), the causes of closure are congenital diseases, residual scarring of leptomeningitides, or tumors of the fourth ventricle. At the level of the basal cisterns and of the subarachnoid spaces of the calvaria, closure can occur after bacterial or parasitic meningitis or tumoral lesions, like in meningiomas of the cranial basis.

Clinical picture

The symptomatology of hydrocephalus varies in relation to the age of the patient at the moment of its clinical manifestation.

The *intrauterine hydrocephalus* is diagnosed with echography. The majority of fetuses also presents other malformations incompatible with life. In fact, two-thirds of the fetuses do not survive the postnatal period long enough to allow treatment of the hydrocephalus and, anyway, the ventricular dilation causes histological changes with serious loss of cerebral tissue and with consequent neurological sequelae.

These considerations have induced neurosurgeons to attempt an early treatment of the hydrocephalus *in utero*. However, attempts at applying a shunt in a human fetus have not been approved, both for technical problems connected with the procedure, and for the high frequency of malformations that notably decrease the vitality of the fetus. It is necessary to consider that a ventricular dilation cannot be evolutive and, therefore, in case of prenatal diagnosis of hydrocephalus, it is recommended to wait until the fetus is vital and to perform a cesarean section. The vitality of the fetus can be determined based on pulmonary maturity, indicated by the lecithin/sphingomyelin ratio in the amniotic fluid.

In *infantile hydrocephalus*, differently from the adult, the clinical manifestations depend on the age of the patient. An expandible skull, with sutures that are still open, allows a considerable ventriculomegaly in absence of symptoms and signs except for a pathological growth of the cranial circumference. In more advanced cases, a clear craniofacial disproportion appears with expansion of the calvaria. The scalp is thin and clear, the veins are congested, the fontanels are stretched and non-pulsating, and the sutures are diastatic. The child is irritable and apathic, feeds with difficulty, and can have a position in opisthotonos. Deficit of conjugated movements of the eyes, disorders of convergence, and downward deviation of ocular globi ("sign of the sun setting") may occur. When the hydrocephalus occurs after closure of the sutures, its clinical characteristics are similar to those of the adult.

The hydrocephalus syndrome in the adult is characterized by signs of endocranial hypertension: headache, vomit, diplopia, upward limitation of the gaze and torpor. If it is not diagnosed, signs of transtentorial and transoccipital herniation occur, with death of the patient.

Diagnosis

The diagnosis of hydrocephalus is based, in addition to clinical anamnestic data, on the instrumental tests: radiography of the skull, echoencephalography, CT, NMR and measuremant of the endocranial pressure.

Radiography of the skull shows diastasis of the sutures, widening of the fontanels, thinning of the calvarial bones, increase of the cranial diameters, disproportion between calvaria and skull base, lowering of the orbital roof, and increase of volume of the posterior cranial fossa in case of Dandy-Walker syndrome.

Echoencephalography shows the dimensions of the ventricles, the thickness of the cortical mantle, the presence of cerebral congenital malformations such as Dandy-Walker cysts, and intraventricular hemorrhages. It is a harmless and easily repeatable test.

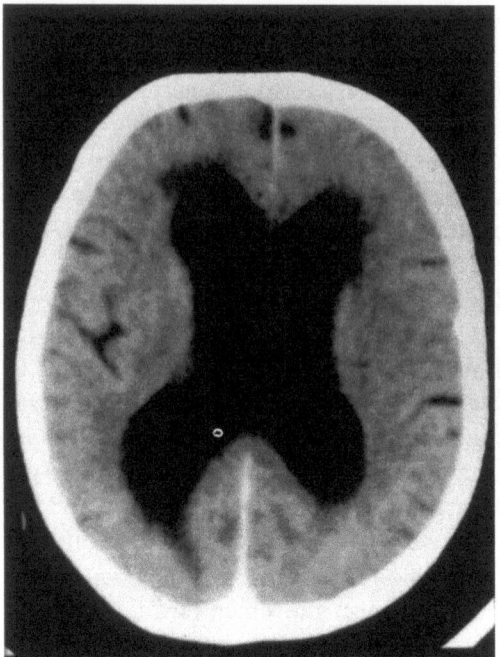

Fig. 6.1. Hydrocephalus. Cerebral CT. Marked dilation of the ventricles with periventricular hypodensity, which is expression of transependymal resorption of cerebrospinal fluid. Reduced subarachnoid spaces of the convexity

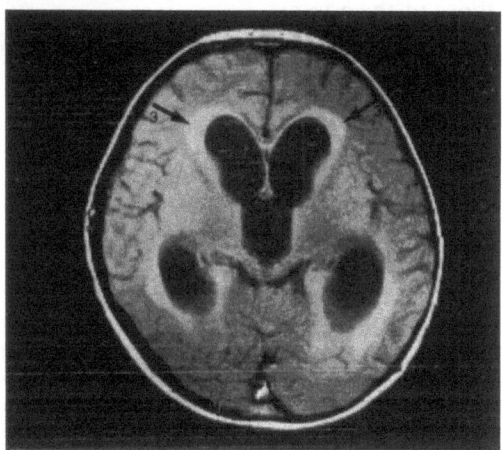

Fig. 6.2. Hydrocephalus. Cerebral CT. Marked dilation of the STVS

CT and *NMR* are the best tests (Figs. 6.1; 6.2) for the evaluation of both suspected and certain hydrocephalus. These tests allow the visualization of the dimensions of the ventricular cavities, the characteristics of the cerebral mantle (thinning of the cerebral mantle under 2.8 cm is usually well endured and does not cause significant growth retardation), the variety of hydrocephalus, the presence of tumoral lesions, aneurysmatic and angiomatous vascular malformations, or cerebral congenital malformations. These tests are also indicated when the shunt does not work properly and for checking the postoperative complications such as subdural hematoma or infection of the ependyma, meninges, and encephalon.

Treatment

In tumoral hydrocephalus, the removal of the tumor is followed, sometimes, by the recanalization of the cerebrospinal pathways with resolution of the hydrocephalus. In other cases, the treatment must resolve the increase of the cerebrospinal pressure. The treatment of hydrocephalus is surgical. However, medical therapies, using drugs like acetazolamide-furosemide, have been attempted to decrease the cerebrospinal fluid production, but with scarce and contrasting results.

Surgical treatment without shunt

In 1918, Dandy described a technique to remove the choroid plexi of the lateral ventricles as a treatment for hydrocephalus. This procedure had poor results because the cerebrospinal fluid continued to be produced by the choroid plexi of the third and fourth ventricles. In 1936, Stookey and Scarff introduced (in cases of triventricular hydrocephalus) the anterior third ventriculostomy by subfrontal approach and puncture of the anterior part of the third ventricle floor at the level of the terminal plate. More recently, *endoscopic ventriculostomy* has been used: a flexible endoscope is introduced in the lateral ventricle via a frontal hole; after visualisation of Monro's foramen, the third ventricle is penetrated and a small fissuration is created, by coagulation, in correspondence of the tuber cinereum. The fissuration is later dilated with a balloon connected to a Fogarty catheter.

Surgical treatment with shunt

In 1939, Torkildsen described a procedure, the posterior ventriculostomy, which allowed the insertion of a tube between the lateral ventricle and cisterna magna for the treatment of obstructive hydrocephalus. Subsequently, other procedures of internal shunt have been suggested. They facilitate the canalization of the sylvian aqueduct, but have given modest results due to the high risk of postoperative deficits.

The external ventricular shunts, instead, have increasingly acquired importance due to the easy application and reliability; ventriculoperitoneal, ventriculo-atrial, and lumboperitoneal shunts are the most used (Figs. 6.3-6.7).

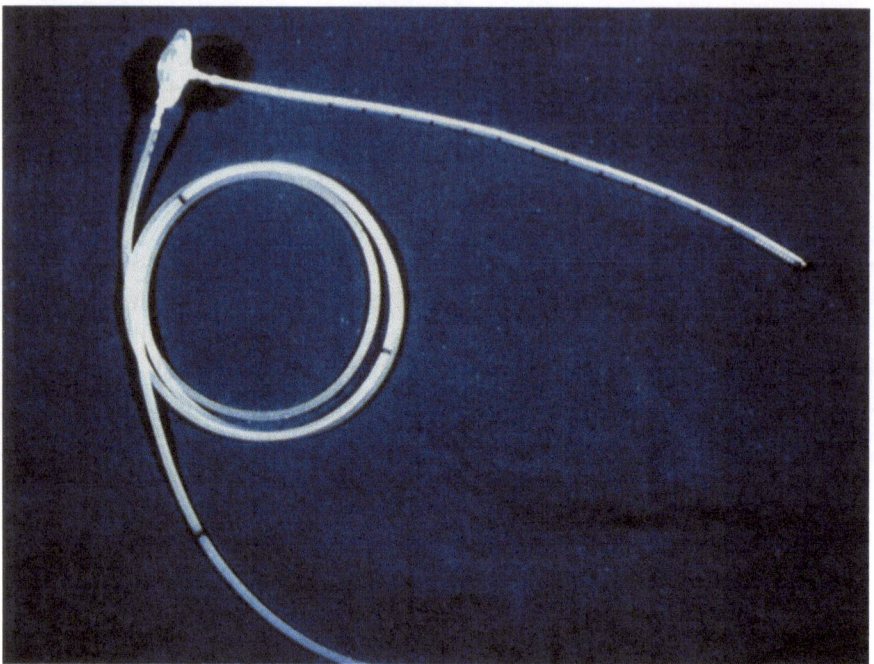

Fig. 6.3. Ventriculoperitoneal Shunt's system

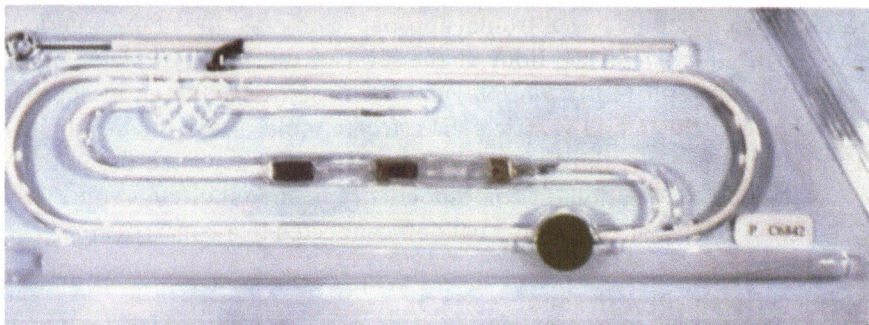

Fig. 6.4. Variable pressure Shunt's system

Complications of the extracranial shunt are: a) *malfunctioning* of the shunt for obstruction of the ventricular or distal catheter, for altered calibration of the valve, for absence of resorption of the cerebrospinal fluid at the level of the outflow organs; b) *infection* of the shunt which occurs in 2%-10% of operated cases (in this case, the diagnosis is facilitated by the presence of signs of sepsis in the meninges or peritoneum, at the systemic

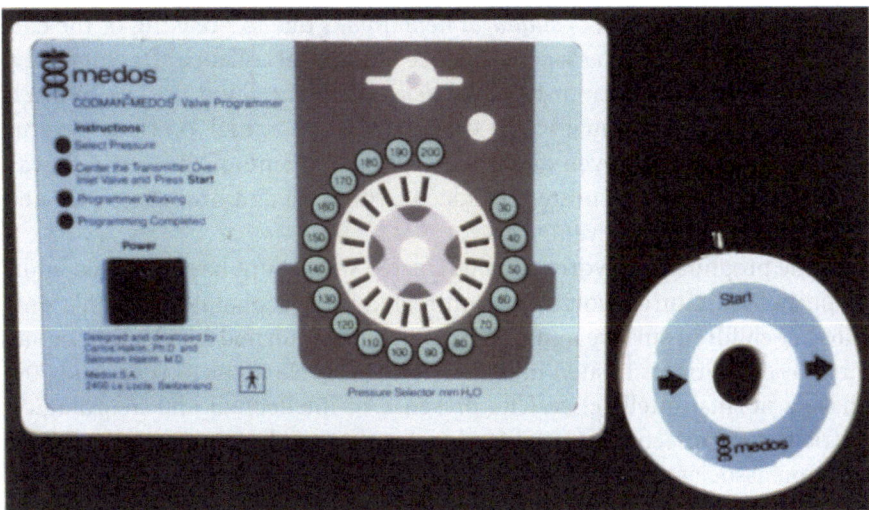

Fig. 6.5. Valve magnetic programmer

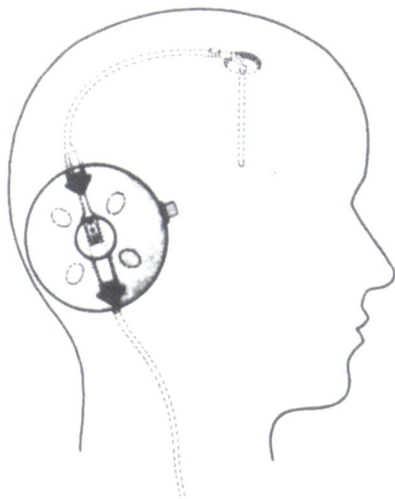

Fig. 6.6. Positioning of a variable pressure Shunt's system

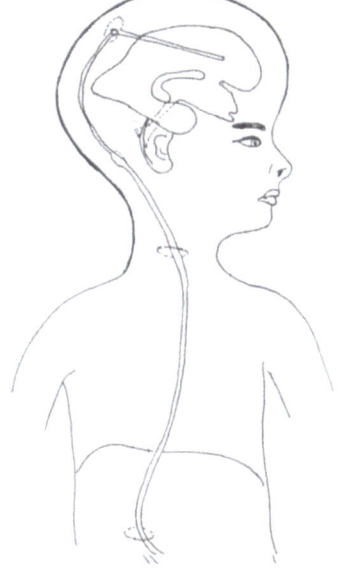

Fig. 6.7. Positioning of the ventriculoperitoneal system

level or in the wound), c) *subdural hematomas* due to breaking of the corticodural bridge veins as a consequence of cerebral collapse after emptying the ventricular cavities; or d) *dependence from the shunt or cleft ventricle syndrome* due, presumably, to the scarce intracranial pressure-volume adaptability, so that even small increases in volume of the ventricle can elicit sudden and intermittent headache, vomiting and drowsiness. CT and NMR show small cleft ventricles.

The prognosis of hydrocephalus treated with shunt has improved enormously. The natural evolution of untreated hydrocephalus shows that only 46% of children survive and only 38% present a normal intellectual capacity. 93% of patients treated in pediatric age survive up to 10 years and 70% have a normal intelligence. The presence of intellectual and neurological deficits can be secondary to infection, intracranial hemorrhage, or malformation associated or not to the hydrocephalus.

Normotensive hydrocephalus

It is a chronic hydrocephalus in which a light gradient of pressure between the ventricles and brain persists. It cause the dilation of the ventricular system. It is mainly observed in elderly patients and it is due to a compromised cerebrospinal circulation at the level of the basal cisterns. It can be the consequence of a cranial trauma, inflammation of the meninges or a subarachnoid hemorrhage. The clinical picture of normal pressure hydrocephalus is characterized by three fundamental symptoms: *psychic disorders* (characterized by progressive mental deterioration until dementia), *urinary incontinence*, and *disorders of gait*. Considering that the characteristic clinical signs of cerebrospinal hypertension are absent, the differential diagnosis includes senile and presenile dementiae and cerebral post-traumatic atrophy. CT and NMR can show a progressive dilation of the ventricular system; unfortunately, this finding cannot be conclusive for a diagnosis of normal pressure hydrocephalus. An important diagnostic test is the measurement of the endocranial pressure by epidural, subdural and intraventricular tubes. This recording highlights, on a tracing of normal intracranial pressure, nocturnal plateaux of increased intracranial pressure of the duration of some minutes up to one or two hours. The treatment of the hydrocephalus gives satisfactory results.

7. Cranioencephalic trauma

The more frequent causes of cranioencephalic trauma are motor accidents, falls, and work or sport accidents. The overall incidence of cranioencephalic trauma is 200 per 100 000 individuals and the average mortality for cerebral lesions is 30 per 100 000 individuals. Studies of the distribution of the incidence in relation to gender and age reveal a male/female ratio of 3:1. Males have an higher incidence than females at all ages, if we exclude very young subjects under 2 years and the elderly over 65 years of age. The highest incidence fluctuates between 15 and 24 years of age.

Classification

A very important classification divides the cranioencephalic trauma in: open trauma and closed trauma.

Open trauma

In open trauma there is a communication between the intracranial space and the external environment. Generally, the trauma is caused by blunt objects or perforating forces which injure the scalp, calvaria and basis of the skull with laceration of the dura mater and encephalon. The open trauma necessitates immediate surgical operation to avoid the onset of intracranial infections and subsequent epileptogenic foci.

Closed trauma

They are provoked by the direct impact with an ample or bevelled surface or by an indirect trauma. If the intensity of the trauma is considerable, it produces fractures and damage to the cerebral parenchyma.

Another distinction to explain the physiopathology of the cranioencephalic injuries is that between direct traumas and indirect traumas.

Direct trauma. The traumatic force hits the head or the head bumps against a fixed obstacle.

Indirect trauma. The brain is affected indirectly by accelerating and decelerating forces, responsible for the sudden displacement of the cerebral parenchyma. An example is the indirect trauma provoked by an abrupt displacement of the shoulders in a child or a fall on the heels or on the pelvis.

Biomechanics

Cranioencephalic trauma is caused by the action of a mechanical load on the cranioencephalic structures. The mechanical load can be: static (rarely) or dynamic.

In the static mechanical load, the traumatic force acts gradually over 200 ms, so that it causes a deformation and crush of the cranial cavity with consequent cerebral compression and cerebral sprain. If the trauma intensity is considerable, it also causes multiple fractures of the skull.

In the dynamic mechanical load, the traumatic force acts over a short time of about 50-100 ms. The dynamic load can be of two types: a) impulsive trauma or trauma by acceleration-deceleration or indirect trauma; or b) trauma by contact or direct impact.

Impulsive trauma or trauma by acceleration-deceleration

Impulsive trauma occurs when the head is mobilized or is sharply stopped without being hit. This situation is observed when the head is moved sharply after a thoracic or facial trauma or after falls on the pelvis or on the heels, or in the case in which a child is seized by the shoulders and shaken with violence. The abrupt movement or arrest of the head produces acceleration and deceleration forces, responsible for brain movements in relation to the dura mater and to the skull, with consequent tension and break of the subdural bridge veins, formation of contusive foci from contrecoup, concussion syndromes and diffuse axonal damage. The damage caused by the impulsive trauma changes in relation to the type of acceleration (translational, rotational, angular), to the intensity, and to the duration and velocity with which the acceleration is applied to the head. Superficial stress affects bridge veins and pial vessels and they produce subdural hematomas, and contrecoup contusions, while deep stress causes the concussion syndrome and diffuse axonal lesions.

Trauma by contact or by impact

The trauma by contact occurs when the head bumps against an obstacle or it is striken by a traumatizing body. The effects of contact trauma are determined both at the level of the impact zone and at a distance, by a folding mechanism of the cranial theca and by the "shock waves". The grevity of those phenomena is in relation to the dimensions of the impact means and to the impact intensity.

Contact trauma with effects on the impact zone

The lesions are in relation to a traumatic force with limited impact surface. When the object (hammer, stone) strikes the skull, it produces an oval sinking in the impact zone and, if the trauma intensity is considerable, a breaking of the table and of the outer cortical (more resistant and elastic). In this way, fractures with radial disposition around the impact zone or depressed fractures are produced.

The fracture can be accompanied by encephalic damage under the impact point, like cerebral laceration or contusion or formation of extradural hematoma due to laceration of the trunk or branches of the middle meningeal artery.

Contact trauma with distance effects

The lesions are in relation to a violent traumatic force and to an ample impact zone (fall with shock on the pavement, shock against the windshield of a car following a collision) which cause a deformation of the skull and the formation of shock waves. The action of the trauma with ample impact zone, if it strikes an area with thick cranial theca, determines a scarce depression or introflexion of the external cortical, while tension waves are formed in the surrounding zone, particularly if the bone has reduced thickness with consequent extroflexion of the inner table and tension of the outer table. If the limits of bone resistance are exceeded, fracture lines form departing from the extroflexion, especially where the tension action prevails, and spread like waves both in the impact zone and along lines of minor resistance, until they involve the base of the skull (linear fractures-fractures of the basis of the skull). The minor resistance zones correspond to the territories included between the pillars (higher resistance zones) which, in number of six, depart from the convexity and go toward the basis of the skull. The shock or tension waves arising from the impact zone can also spread across the brain, extending to the opposite side, or they can be amplified and reverberated inside the brain. If the intensity of the shock waves overcomes the brain resistance, cerebral parenchyma and vessel damage (axonal lesions, diffuse lesions of the microcircle with loss of autoregulation, hypoxic and ischemic lesions) will occur in areas distant from the impact site (contrecoup lesions).

The frontobasal lesions are typical of this mechanism, they are secondary to occipital trauma and due to the movement of the frontal lobes on the bony roughness of the anterior cranial fossa. Temporal injuries due to occipital shock are also typical. They are secondary to contracoup injuries on the lesser wing of the sphenoid bone.

Physiopathology

The pathological alterations caused by closed cranial traumas can be classified into two types:
1) Focal or primary lesions
2) Secondary lesions
   - Metabolic lesions by hypoxia and ischemia
   - Diffuse lesions of the microcircle due to loss of autoregulation
   - Diffuse axonal lesion

Focal or primary lesions

Generally, the focal lesions occur under the site of the trauma and they are due to the mechanical action of the traumatic forces on the underlying tissues and structures. The most common focal lesions are: lesions of the soft tissues, cranial fractures, extra-intradural and parenchymal haemorrhages, cranial nerves lesions, contusions, encephalic contusion and encephalic necrosis.

Secondary lesions

Metabolic lesions by hypoxia and ischemia

The cerebral metabolism is exclusively aerobic. The cerebral oxygen consumption (the brain constitutes 2% of body weight) is about 20% of the total oxygen consumed by the entire organism. Therefore, the brain is more sensitive than other organs to hypoxia and anoxia. In cranial traumas, a decreased oxygen tension can be caused by deficient blood oxygenation due to peripheral or central causes or due to decreased cerebral blood flow (critical value, < 30 ml/100 g per minute) caused by shock, hypotension, anemia, cardiac insufficiency, or intracranial hypertension.

Among the peripheral causes responsible for insufficient supply of oxygen, we find:

– Alterations at the thoracic level (pleuropulmonary injuries with hemopneumothorax, costal and diaphragmatic lesions).
– Alterations at the upper airway level (tracheobronchial obstruction by regurgitated blood after vomiting, foreign bodies, tongue fall in the retropharynx in patients with loss of consciousness).

Among the central causes we find brainstem damage for direct or indirect (concussion) action. The decreased or absent oxygen and glucose supply to the nervous cells forces their metabolism to switch from aerobic to anaerobic, activating a cascade of biochemal and vascular phenomena, which severely damage the nervous cells. The oxygen and glucose deficit leads to an accumulation of lactic acid, with consequent lactic acidosis. This accelerates and increases the ischemic process by vasospasm, altering the calcium metabolism by accumulation of Ca^{++} and Na^+ inside the cell and exit of K^+.

The altered biochemical mechanisms release metabolites, like prostaglandin E2 and thromboxane, capable of inducing vasospasm, thrombosis and edema.

Additionally, during the precocious phase of the hypoxic-ischemic stress of the nervous tissue, oxygen free radicals are released, causing tissular damage by reacting with the cellular components.

Diffuse lesions by microcircle due to loss of autoregulation

After cranial trauma, we can have diffuse damage of the microcircle with precocious cerebrovascular autoregulation loss and decreased response to the changes of CO_2 levels. The autoregulation loss makes the brain particularly sensitive to changes of the systemic arterial pressure, so that an eventual pressure increase can cause hyperemia, cerebral edema and hemorrhagic foci, while a pressure decrease can aggravate the ischemic damage.

After cranial trauma, the alteration of the autoregulation mechanism at the level of the microcircle and the metabolic injuries by hypoxia and ischemia are also responsible for brain edema. Brain edema consists of an increase of the extravascular liquid compartment of the brain. From a physiopathological point of view, the edema can be divided in: cellular or cytotoxic edema and vasogenic edema.

Cytotoxic edema is caused by the alteration of membrane permeability of the nervous cells due to the altered regulation of Na, K, and Ca pumps, with consequent intracellular liquid accumulation. Cytotoxic edema involves, mainly, the astrocytes of the gray matter; this swelling phenomenon can damage the nervous cell in an irreversible way.

Vasogenic edema is the consequence of ischemic or biochemical stress or damage to the cerebral vessels which involves the membrane of the endothelial cells of the capillary wall.

Diffuse axonal injury

This term describes a post-traumatic, prolonged coma, not caused by masses (hematoma, contusion) or by ischemic lesions. The trauma involves a group of axons of the corpus callosum, brainstem and periventricular area. The transport of materials from the cell body to the nerve endings is interrupted by axotomy, with consequent accumulation and axonal edema. The increased membrane permeability allows the passage and accumulation of macromolecules like proteins or other solutes or liquids into the extracellular space. The vasogenic edema mainly affects the white substance. The association of cytotoxic and vasogenic edema causes an increase of the cerebral volume, intracranial hypertension, decrease of the cerebral perfusion and metabolic alteration of the nervous cells.

Clinical picture

The symptomatology of cranioencephalic trauma changes in relation to the type of lesion caused by the trauma.

Soft tissue injuries

Excoriation: contused injury with epidermis involvement up to the dermis;

contusion: injury caused by a blunt object, it is characterized by hematic infiltration of the scalp; it occurs like a swelling at the level of the traumatized area;

wound: solution of continuity involving skin, hypoderm and the inferior anatomical layers; it can be simple, stellate and/or with substance loss in relation to the traumatizing agent;

lacero-contused wound: to the solution of continuity are added injuries caused by bruising and traction forces, therefore the margins are irregular and anfractuous;

subcutaneous hematoma: blood collection between skin and galea;

subgaleal hematoma: blood collection between galea and pericranium;

cephalo-hematoma: blood collection between periost and bone. This is found almost exclusively during the neonatal period and it appears like a deeply localized mass in the scalp; the most frequent location is the parietal region.

Cranial fractures

The cranial fractures, in relation to their location, are distinguished into fractures of the calvaria and fractures of the skull base. In relation to their morphology they are distinguished into linear, depressed, and growing fractures (Figs. 7.1-7.4).

Linear fractures: represent about the 80% of the cranial fractures and are the result of a major cranial trauma. Generally, they do not require a specific treatment (Figs. 7.5; 7.6).

Depressed fractures: are fractures in which one or more osseous fragments are driven within the cranial cavity. They can cause dural and cerebral lacerations with possible neurological deficit and formation of epileptogenic foci.

Growing fractures (Fig. 7.7): are linear or depressed fractures which grow with time. For their formation, a dural or arachnoid break is necessary, with consequent formation of subgaleal, pulsating CSF accumulation. This causes a progressive increase of the bony discontinuity. They are characteristic in children under 8 years of age.

Clinically, they appear like a pulsating cranial defect. The fractures can occur with spontaneous pain or induced pain by palpation on the lesion site, with extra- and intracerebral hemorrhages, with cerebral lacero-bruising foci and with cranial nerve deficits.

Among the complications of the cranial basis fractures, we find CSF fistulas, pneumoencephalon and septic processes.

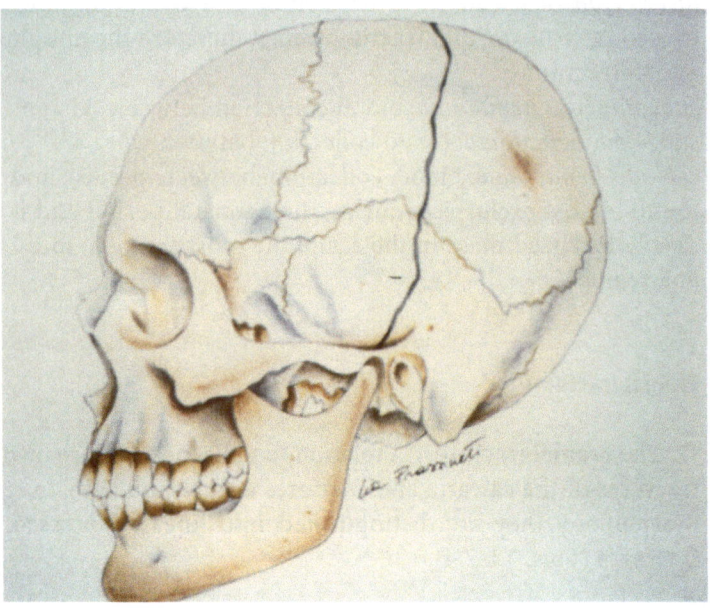

Fig. 7.1. Parietotemporal linear fractures

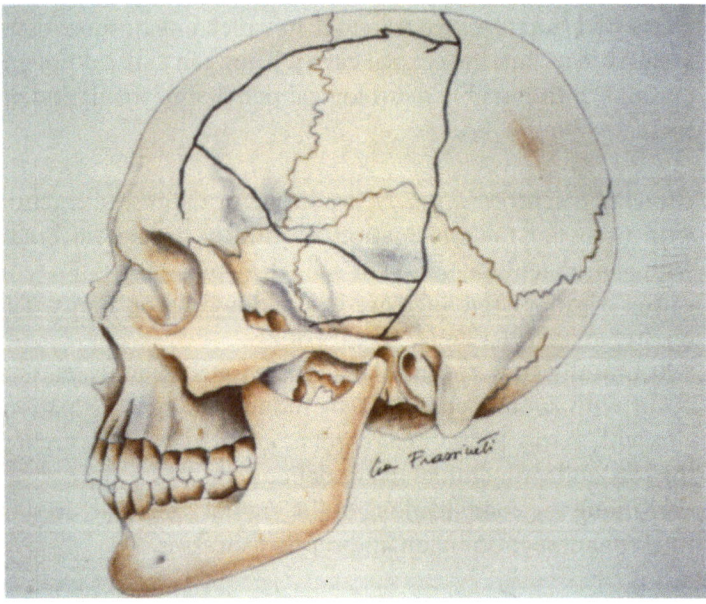

Fig. 7.2. Parietotemporal "burst" linear fractures

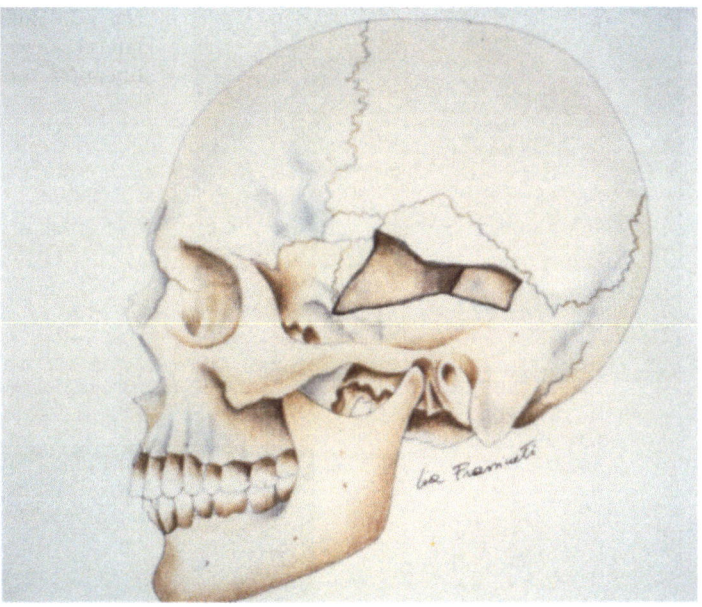

Fig. 7.3. Temporal depressed fracture

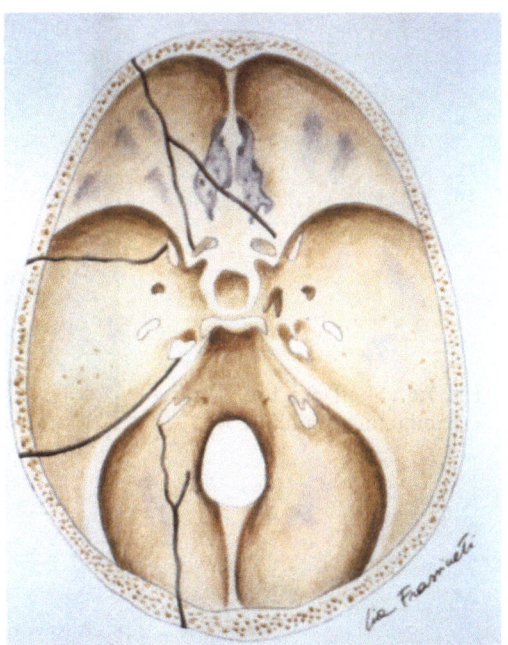

Fig. 7.4. Trajectories of the cranial vault fractures radiating
toward the cranial basis

112   Essential illustrated neurosurgery

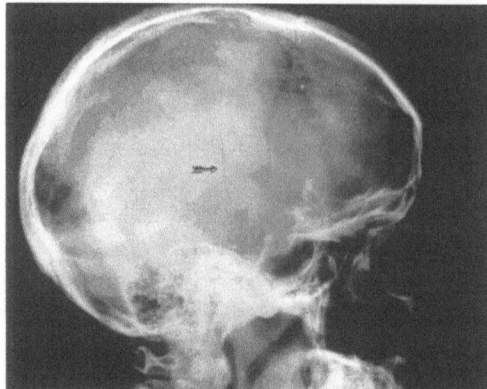

Fig. 7.5. Skull fracture. X-ray, lateral view. Temporoparietal linear fracture

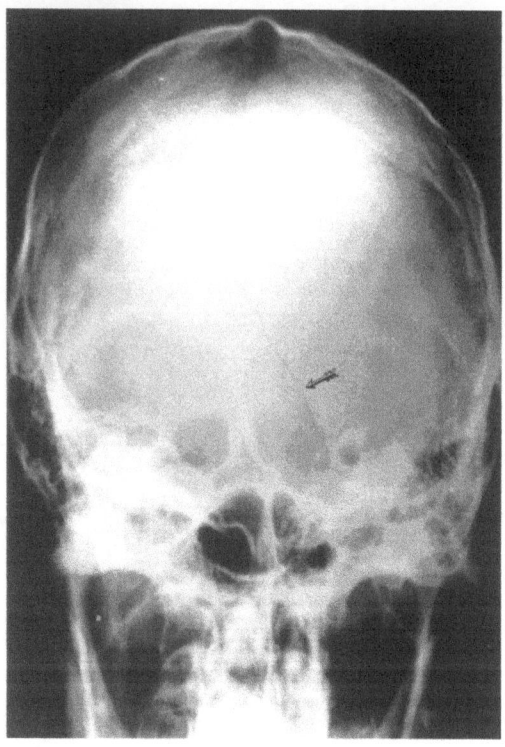

Fig. 7.6. Skull fracure. X-ray. Occipital linear fracture

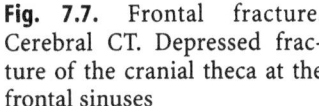

Fig. 7.7. Frontal fracture. Cerebral CT. Depressed fracture of the cranial theca at the frontal sinuses

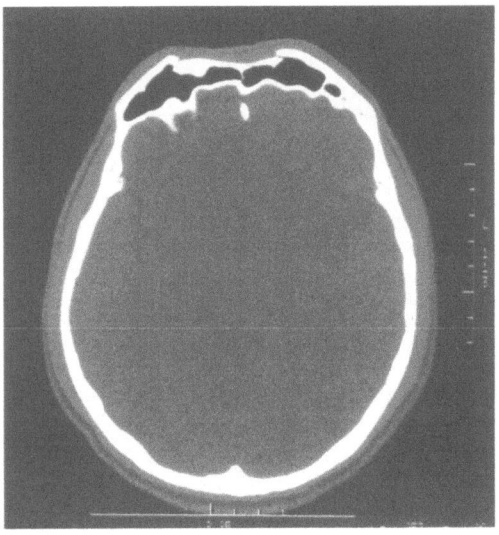

Extracerebral lesions

Epidural hematoma

It is a hematic collection between the inner table and the dura mater; it can be arterial (often due to breaking of the middle meningeal artery or of its branch), venous (breaking of a venous sinus or dural veins), or arterio-venous (Figs. 7.8; 7.9).

The most frequent localizations are temporoparietal and temporo-fronto-parietal. It is rare in elderly persons, due to the tenacious dural adherence to the inner table, and during the first years of life.

The hematoma occurs during the first 48 hours in 75% of cases, and 1-2 days after trauma in 25% of cases.

The clinical signs depend on the velocity of growth of the hematoma and the presence of intradural injuries.

The patient, after a cranial trauma, can present different states of consciousness: a) the patient loses consciousness for a minute or an hour, then becomes conscious and then unconscious again; b) the patient is, initially, conscious and lucid but progressively loses connection with the environment; or c) the patient, after the trauma, remains unconscious. Afterwards, the clinical signs of the hematoma are due to the intracranial hypertension (e.g. headache, vomiting, psychomotorial agitation, confusional state, drowsiness, increase of the systemic arterial pressure, and bradycardia), tentorial herniation of the temporal lobe (homolateral anisocoria, ingravescent hemiparesis and positive Babinsky's sign, contralateral to the

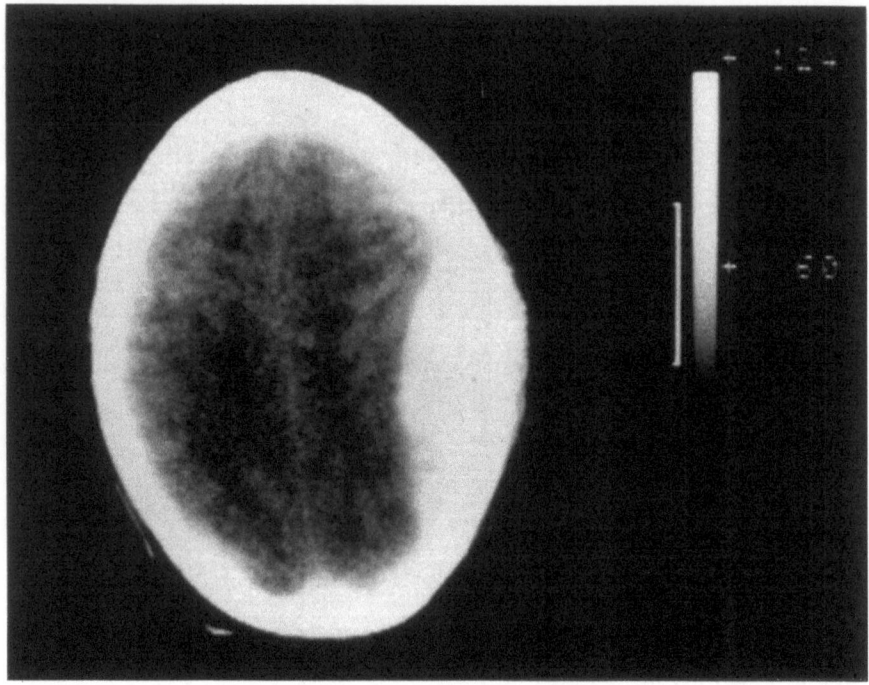

Fig. 7.8. Epidural hematoma. Cerebral CT. Right frontoparietal epidural hematic collection

hematoma), hemiplegia, bilateral mydriasis, and vegetative disorders, culminating with death for bulbar paralysis.

Subdural hematoma

It is a blood collection between the dura mater and the subarachnoid space. The hemorrhage is due to breaking of the cortico-dural veins, of the venous dural sinuses or of the cortical vessels after lesions of the cerebral surface.

In relation to the time elapsed between trauma and clinical signs, hematomas are distinguish into: a) acute (appearance within 48-72 hours); b) sub-acute (appearance within 3-20 days); or c) chronic (appearance from 3 weeks to some months).

Acute subdural hematoma

The symptomatology depends on the intensity of the trauma and the severity of concomitant lesions of the cerebral parenchyma (Fig. 7.10).

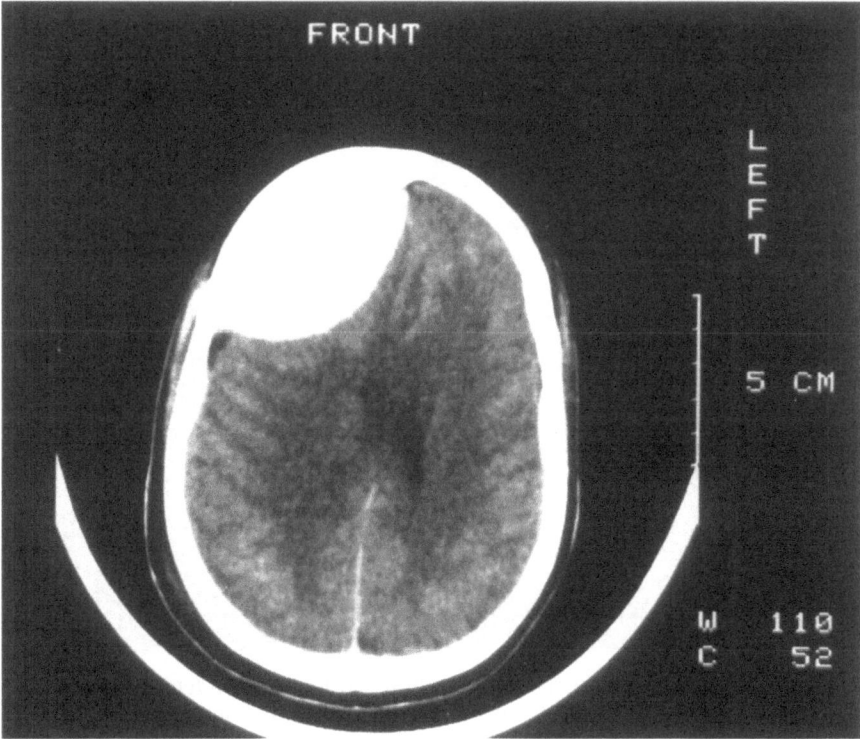

Fig. 7.9. Epidural hematoma. Cerebral CT. Right frontohematic collection with biconvex morphology lens, with compression on the inferior cerebral parenchyma

The highest incidence has been found between 40 and 50 years of age, being quite rare before 20 years.

We can distinguish three clinical varieties in relation to the evolution of the state of consciousness: 1) a patient, suffering a light or modest trauma, can remain conscious or lose consciousness for a short time (a few minutes to one hour), then remain lucid for a few minutes to hours and become again somnolent and soporous, until falling into a coma; 2) the patient, after a cranial trauma of medium intensity, remains in a coma for a short time (a few minutes to one hour), then regains contact with the environment, remaining lucid or confused with psychomotor agitation and then presents again worsening of the state of consciousness until coma; or 3) the patient, after a cranial trauma of considerable intensity, remains in a coma.

While the state of consciousness has a varying behavior, the neurological state, during the hours following the accident, can worsen in a progressive and uniform way. Signs of intracranial hypertension (headache, vom-

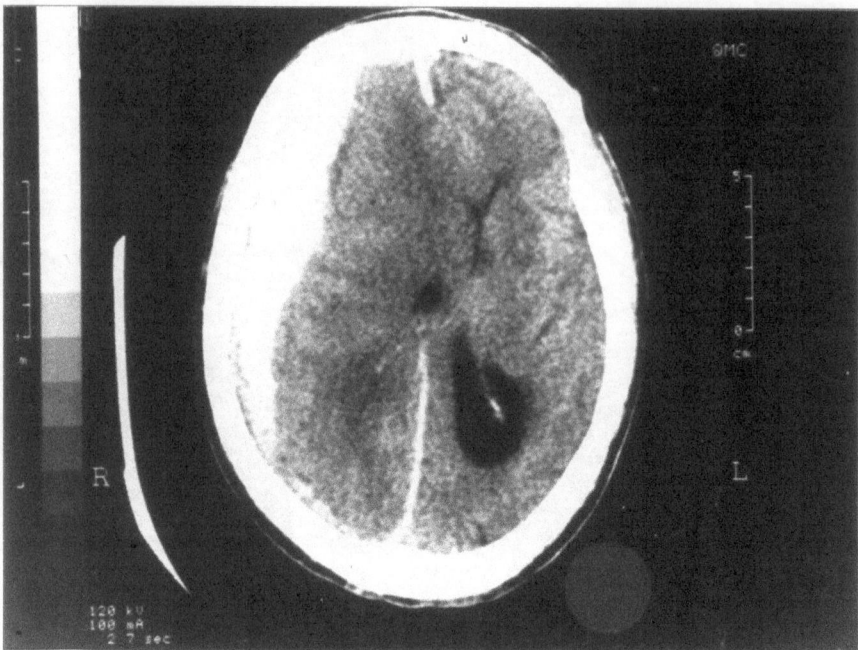

Fig. 7.10. Acute subdural hematoma. Cerebral CT. Right frontotemporal, extensive hematic collection with morphology at flap localized in frontotemporal site, with compression of the right lateral ventricle and contralateral displacement of the controlateral STVS

iting, psychomotorial agitation, increased arterial systemic pressure and concomitant bradycardia) appear first, followed by signs of compression of the brainstem by tentorial herniation of the temporal lobe (homolateral mydriasis, hemiparesis with contralateral Babinsky's sign), decerebration signs, bilateral mydriasis, and severe vegetative disorders until death for bulbar paralysis.

Subacute subdural hematoma (Fig. 7.11)

The highest incidence is observed in patients over 40-50 years of age; it is rare in children.

In relation to the evolution of the state of consciousness, we can distinguish two clinical varities:

a) The patient, after a cranial trauma of modest entity, remains conscious or loses consciousness for a few minutes. After a few days of well being, he laments about headache, and is confused, slackened, and somnolent. Focal signs appear (e.g. hemiparesis, language disorders, alterations of the visual field), together with signs of intracranial hypertension and

Fig. 7.11. Subacute subdural hematoma. MRI, T1-weighted image, coronal view. Subdural hematic collection in the right hemispheric area with compression on the inferior cerebral parenchyma

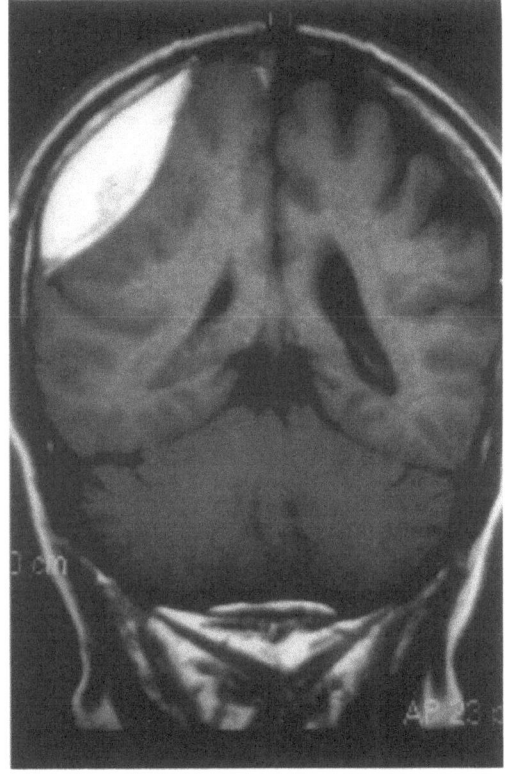

transtentorial herniation of the temporal lobe. If the diagnosis is not immediately effected the patient dies for bulbar paralysis.

b) The patient, after a trauma of middle intensity, remains in a coma for some hours or days, then regains contact with the environment but remains somnolent, confused, and agitated. After a few days, there is a worsening of the condition: periods of stupor or superficial coma alternate with phases of lucidity. At the same time, focal deficits worsen or appear, together with signs of intracranial hypertension and tentorial herniation of the temporal lobe. The patient dies of bulbar paralysis if a surgical operation to remove the hematoma is not performed.

Chronic subdural hematoma

It is an encapsulated accumulation of liquid, of a dark brown or yellow color, formed by water and degraded blood, growing gradually (Fig. 7.12). The increase in volume is due to a process of fluidification of the hematoma and to the lysis of the cellular components, which increases protein concentration and osmolarity.

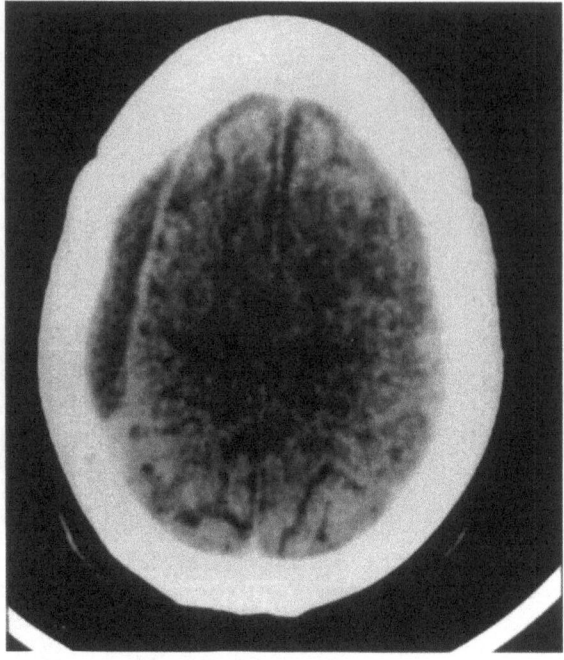

Fig. 7.12. Chronic subdural hematoma. Hypodense and dyshomogeneous area localized in the subdural right frontoparietal side with hematic components

The capsule, acting as an osmotic membrane, allows the liquoral diffusion within the hematoma with consequent increases in volume.

A repeated hemorrhage from the neoformed vessels of the hematoma membrane can also contribute to the increase in volume.

Symptomatology. The chronic subdural hematoma is more frequent during adult age and in elderly patients. The signs are variable and not always pathognomonic.

The symptomatology starts in an insidious way and, in elderly patients, can be mistaken for a demential syndrome (decreased critical capacity, attention and memory disorders, apathy, confusional state, affectivity alteration) or cerebrovascular syndrome (sensorimotor deficit). Rarely, it can occur with a focal or generalized epileptic crisis. If it is not diagnosed, signs of intracranial hypertension, transtentorial herniation with stress of the brainstem, and vegetative disorders will appear, until death.

Subarachnoid hemorrhage

This is an accumulation of blood in the subarachnoid space due to breaking of corticopial vessels at the level of the superficial lacero-bruising foci.

The presence of blood in the subarachnoid space irritates the meninges, increases the osmotic tension in the cerebrospinal fluid, and alters of the cerebrospinal fluid circulation.

Symptomatology. When the subarachnoid hemorrhage is not accompanied by other concomitant extracerebral (extra- and subdural hematomas) and cerebral (cerebral hematomas, lacero-bruising foci, diffuse edema) lesions, the symptomatology is characterized by signs of meningeal reaction (headache, stiff neck after the first 24 hours, flexed lower limbs), psychic disorders (apathy, restlessness, psychomotor agitation, attention disorders, drowsiness), and hyperthermia. If the amount of blood in the subarachnoid space is considerable and blocks the cerebrospinal fluid circulation or resorption, signs of intracranial hypertension due to hydrocephalus will appear.

Cranial nerve lesions

A trauma of medium and strong intensity can lead to contusion, laceration, or tearing of the cranial nerves, especially when the trauma causes fractures of the cranial basis.

Deficits of the optic nerve, chiasm and olfactory nerve are present in patients affected by traumas of the frontal region. Deficit of cranial nerve III is more frequently due to transtentorial herniation of the temporal lobe. Deficit of the cranial nerve VII-VIII is due to longitudinal fractures of the petrous part of the temporal bone.

Intracerebral lesions

Intracerebral hematoma

It is collection of blood limited to the cerebral parenchyma. A trauma which causes intracerebral hematoma is of strong intensity and is accompained by loss of consciousness. The areas most frequently affected are the temporal regions and, more rarely, the frontal, parietal, or cerebellar regions.

Symptomatology. The symptoms of the intracerebral hematoma are not pathognomonic, and can be confused with other expansive intracranial lesions and with extracerebral hematic accumulation (extradural and subdural hematomas). The symptoms and signs depend on the localization and volume of the hematoma: deterioration of consciousness, focal deficit, and signs of intracranial hypertension.

Lacero-contused foci

They are represented by zones of the brain with hemorrhagic and necrotic areas. Generally, they are multiple and localized at the impact site or, more frequently, distant from it (Fig. 7.13). The areas most frequently affected are the temporal and frontal lobes.

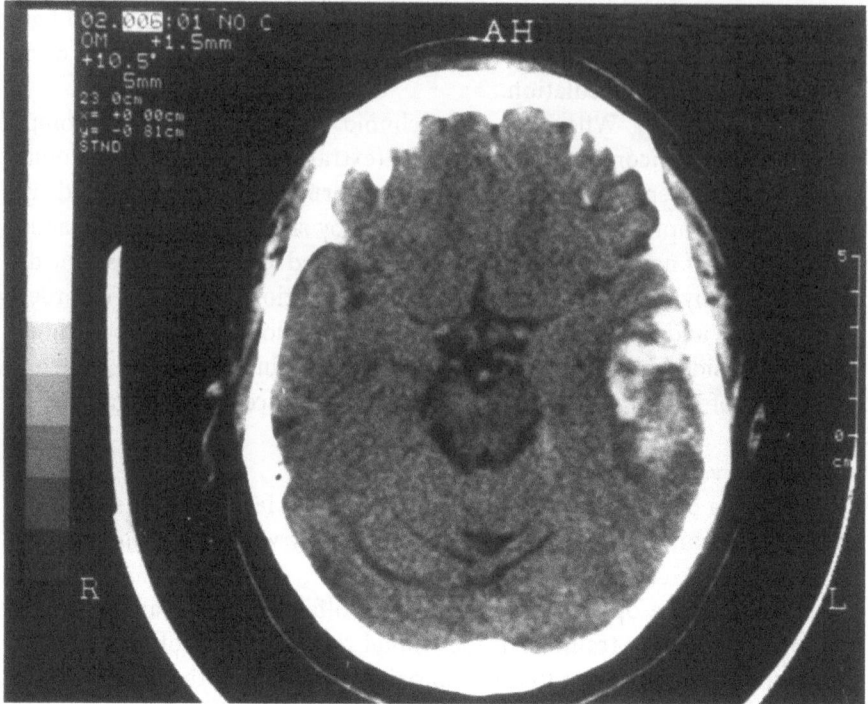

Fig. 7.13. Brain contusion. Cerebral CT. Left temporal contusion. Dyshomogeneous density with large nuclei of hematic infarction

Symptomatology. The symptoms change in relation to the dimension and location of the primary lesion and to the type of associated lesions.

We can observe: consciousness alterations, irritative focal signs, deficit signs, symptoms of intracranial hypertension, signs of transtentorial herniation with stress of the brainstem, vegetative disorders and finally exitus.

Post-traumatic intracranial complications

They consist of cerebrospinal dura fistula, carotid-cavernous fistula, pneumoencephalon, hydrocephalus, subdural higroma, and meningitis.

Cerebrospinal dura fistula
   This is a pathological communication between the subarachnoid space and the external environment due to interruption of the meningeal and osseous envelopes. When the fracture involves the posterior cranial fossa

and/or the paranasal sini, there is an outflow of cerebrospinal fluid from the nasal fossae, called cerebrospinal rhinorrhea. If the fracture affects the petrousa and is associated with laceration of the tympanic membrane, there is outflow of cerebrospinal fluid from the external acoustic canal, called cerebrospinal otorrhea.

The incidence of liquorrhea in patients with cranial trauma is about 2%. Usually it occurs within 24 hours of trauma, sometimes after some weeks, rarely after some months.

The quantity of cerebrospinal fluid can vary from a few drops a day to a conspicuous and continuous loss. Usually, it is omolateral to the side of the fracture.

In about 70% of cases it regresses spontaneously due to granulation and healing phenomena or to herniation of the brain at the level of the dural and osseous discontinuity.

The liquorrhea occurs with cerebrospinal fluid loss, with focal signs related to the fracture location (anosmia, hypoacusis, visual and campimetric deficits, carotid-cavernous fistula), with headache in cases of considerable loss of cerebrospinal fluid (cerebrospinal hypotension) or, when an aerocele is present, with intracranial hypertension signs or meningitis in cases of septic complications.

The diagnosis for the localization of the fistulous connection is based on radiographical and computed tomographical visualization of the cranial basis. CT cisternography, using radiopaque substances (metrizamide) injected in the subarchnoid space by a lumbar puncture or markers (fluorescin) injected in the cerebrospinal fluid, is especially revealing. The examination with radioisotopes (labeled albumin) is useful in case a fistula is present.

The treatment for traumatic liquorrhea, not regressing spontaneously, is surgical and consists in repairing the dural and osseous discontinuity.

The operation is effected after a period of about 12-15 days from the onset of the cerebrospinal fluid loss. During this waiting period the patient is protected with an antibiotic therapy at very high dosage.

Carotid-cavernous fistula

It is an anomalous communication between the cavernous sinus and the intracavernous tract of the carotid artery. It is determined by a violent cranial trauma in the frontal or orbital areas. From the wall of the fissured carotid artery, arterial blood blends with venous blood of the cavernous sinus. An increase of flow and pressure is determined in the venous sinus, with consequent engorgement and inversion of the circulation at the level of the efferent venous vessels.

Symptomatology. Symptoms can appear immediately after the trauma or after some time, from weeks to months. The symptoms include: pulsating exophthalmos (synchronous with the cardiac activity), conjunctival chemosis, corneal alterations, visual loss secondary to the damage of the optic nerve or the retina due to insufficient blood supply or to ocular hypertension (glaucoma), and deficit of the cranial nerves III, IV and VI due to compression of the cavernous sinus.

Subjectively, the patient perceives an intracranial murmur, synchronous with the pulse. This can also be perceived by the examiner placing a phonendoscope on the eyeball.

The diagnosis is made both by clinical examination and angiography of the carotid artery, which shows the signs of arteriovenous communication in the cavernous sinus revealed by the opacification of the cavernous sinus, superior ophthalmic vein, sphenoparietal sinus, intracavernous sinus, and superior petrous sinus (Fig. 7.14a,b).

CT with contrast medium shows a dilation of the cavernous sinus and injection of pathologic drain veins.

NMR has a specific application for the study of this pathology, giving the best spatial documentation of the involved vascular structures and, in some cases, showing the site of formation of the fistula. NMR, at the level of the hypertrophic cavernous sinus, shows a zone of absent signal in all of the available sequences (T1-PD-T2) due to the high velocity flow established inside the sinus itself. This appearence is also well evident at the level of the hypertrophic ophthalmic vein.

Therapy consists in the closure of the fistulous connection between the carotid artery and cavernous sinus. This closure can be obtained: a) with an inflatable microballoon, with platinum coils, or by embolization with acrylic material, b) with surgical procedure, by opening the cavernous sinus and closing the discontinuity of the intracavernous carotid artery or with the obliteration of the cavernous sinus by Surgicel or other materials.

Pneumocephalon

The word "pneumocephalon" means presence of air in the cranial cavity. It can be localized in the extradural space (rarely), or the subdural, subarachnoid or intraventricular spaces. Generally it is associated with liquorrhea.

This complication occurs when trauma causes cranial fracture and tearing of the dura mater at the same time, with consequent communication between cranial cavity and external environment. Usually, it is a consequence of frontal fractures with involvement of the frontal sinuses and of the cribiform plate.

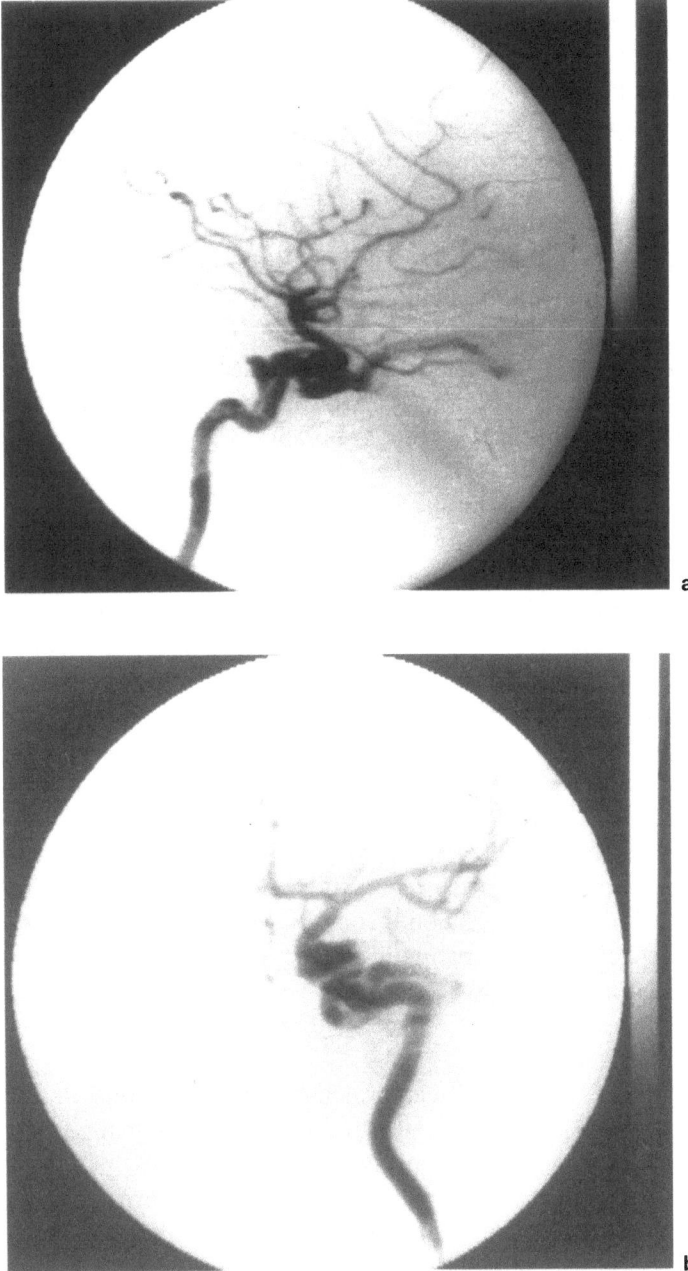

Fig. 7.14a,b. Carotid-cavernous fistula. Digital arterial angiography, lateral (a) and anteroposterior (b) views. Contrast medium in the cavernous sinus. Marked dilation of the ophthalmic vein and hypertrophy of the ophthalmic artery

The presence of air in the cranial cavity can produce: hypertensive pneumocephalon and non-hypertensive pneumocephalon.

In case of hypertensive pneumocephalons at the level of the osteo-dural discontinuity, a valve mechanism is established: during efforts, cough, sneezes, and nose blowing. Air enters but can not outflow, leading to intracranial hypertension.

The symptomatology of pneumocephalon is various; in case of non-hypertensive pneumocephalon, the only symptom can be headache; in case of hypertensive pneumocephalon we may observe: a) frontal psychic syndrome (apathy, disinterestedness, slackening, drowsiness); b) intracranial hypertension syndrome (headache, vomiting, arterial hypertension, bradycardia, signs of transtentorial herniation, decerebration signs, and vegetative disorders until death for bulbar paralysis).

A very serious complication is meningitis, secondary to penetration of germs across the osteo-dural discontinuity.

The diagnosis is based on the plain radiographic films, which show the presence of intracranial air and the rimae of fracture, generally involving the frontal sinus and cribriform plate of the ethmoid bone.

CT allows the visualization, besides big pneumocephalus, of small collection of air and, in particular, the fistulous connection at the level of the osseous discontinuity (Fig. 7.15).

NMR clearly shows the presence of air in the cranial cavity. In fact, the air sacs appear as areas of complete absence of signal in contrast to the cerebrospinal fluid in all the sequences (especially in T1 and T2).

Surgical treatment is necessary in hypertensive pneumocephalon to decompress the brain and to repair the osseo-dural discontinuity. In non-hypertensive pneumocephalon, generally, we have spontaneous recovery due to the closure of the fistulous connection by blood clots, teared brain tissue and granulation tissue.

Subdural hygroma

It is an accumulation of cerebrospinal fluid, of normal appearance or slighty xanthochromic, in the subdural space. We can distinguish two varieties: acute hygroma and chronic hygroma.

Acute hygroma is a subdural accumulation of cerebrospinal fluid due to laceration of the arachnoid membrane through which the cerebrospinal fluid comes out and remains trapped in the subdural space. If the lacerated tissue creates a valve mechanism, only allowing the passage of the cerebrospinal fluid in the subdural space, we have a progressive accumulation of fluid and increase in volume of the hygroma.

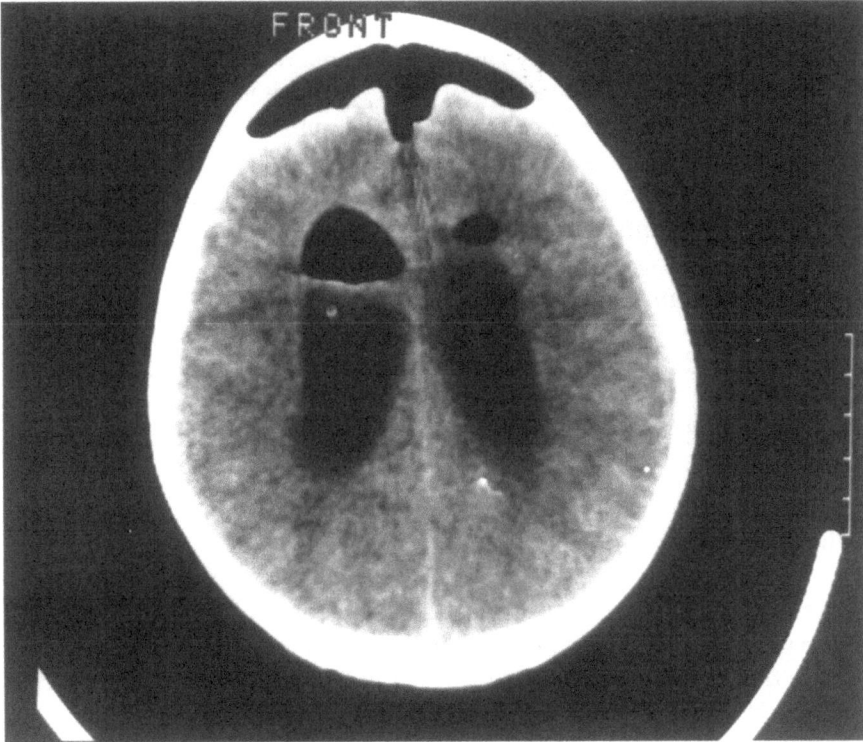

Fig. 7.15. Post-traumatic pneumoencephalo. Cerebral CT. Extensive aerial collection at the level of the anterior part of the lateral ventricle medium cells and bilaterally at the level of the frontal subarachnoid spaces

Chronic hygroma is a rare form, whose pathogenesis is essentially similar to that of the chronic subdural hematoma.

The symptomatology is characterized by headache, vomiting, psychic slackening, sleepiness, hemiparesis contralateral to the lesion, signs of transtentorial herniation, reaction of decerebration, disorders of the vegetative functions, and death for bulbar paralysis.

The diagnosis is based on the clinical picture and cerebral CT. CT shows the presence of a hypodense accumulation similar to cerebrospinal fluid, which coats part or all of the hemisphere, contralateral shift from the midline of the ventricular structures, and disappearance or decrease of the subarachnoid spaces on the side of the cerebrospinal fluid collection.

The therapy is surgical and consists in removal of the hygroma by drilling a hole and opening the dura mater.

Post-traumatic hydrocephalus

It consists of an abnormal increase of the ventricular, cerebrospinal fluid under pressure. From a clinical point of view, it is useful to distinguish the post-traumatic hydrocephalus into acute, subacute and chronic forms.

The pathogenesis is represented by an obstacle to the cerebrospinal fluid flow from clots present along cerebrospinal fluid pathways: Monro's foramina, third ventricle, sylvian aqueduct, fourth ventricle, cisterns of the cranial basis and calvaria.

The symptomatology is characterized by symptoms of intracranial hypertension.

The treatment consists in the application of a shunt which allows the outflow of the cerebrospinal fluid from the ventricles to an extracranial cavity (e.g. abdomen, heart, ureter) or into the intracranial cisterns.

Diagnostic iter

An attentive and systematic assessment of the neurological conditions of the patient affected by cranio-encephalic trauma is necessary for the choice of the diagnostic procedures which will indicate the appropriate surgical approach.

The neurological evaluation should include the state of consciousness, motor response, characteristics of the pupils, ocular movements, and vegetative signs.

State of consciousness

The grades of alteration of consciousness are various, from torpor to stupor and coma. Torpor is a state of reduction of vigilance and mental activity which causes drowsiness and psychomotor excitation with a confusional status. Stupor is a condition of "non-response" from which the subject cannot be awakened.

The trauma can cause memory alterations, such as retrograde amnesia (memory loss of events which happened before the trauma) or anterograde amnesia (memory loss of events which happened after the trauma).

Motor response

The evaluation of the motor response is in relation to the capacity of the patient to collaborate with the examiner. In a patient who collaborates, the motor response can be scored according to five grades.

The evaluation of a patient who does not collaborate, or is in a coma, is based on the observation of the response to external nociceptive stimuli.

We can observe: a) absence of response; b) response in flexion or decortication (adduction and retraction of the shoulders, flexion of the elbows and hands, the lower limbs can be flexed or extended), and c) response in extension or decerebration (head and neck in extension, upper and lower limbs in extension, condition of opisthotonos).

Pupils

The repeated observation of the pupils is of great importance. In fact, the variation of their dimensions and reactivity represents a possible and initial sign of worsening of the state of consciousness.

A monolateral progressive dilation indicates the possible formation of a voluminous lesion (hematomas, cerebral lacero-contused foci) with tentorial herniation. This causes paralysis of the third cranial nerve which contains pupillomotor fibers.

Bilateral mydriatic pupils are expression of a mesencephalic lesion and represent a late sign of tentorial herniation, with negative prognosis.

Pupils in an intermediate position, irregular and not reactive, are expression of a lesion localized at the mesencephalic level due to compression of the descending sympathetic and parasympathetic fibers.

Small and reactive pupils (miosis) are sign of a diencephalic injury.

Punctiform pupils like a "pin head" (miosis), are expression of tegmental lesions of the pons due to interruption of the sympathethic pathways.

Monolateral miosis with enophthalmos and modest lid ptosis is sign of the Bernard–Horner syndrome, caused by a lesion to the sympathetic system descending from the hypothalamus to the bulb or at cervical level.

Movements of ocular globi

The conjugated deviation of the eyes on the horizontal plane is expression of a homolateral hemispheric lesion (frontal or occipital) or of a contralateral pontine lesion. The non-conjugated ocular deviation with the ocular globi positioned on different axes indicates a lesion at the level of the brainstem. The down-ward conjugated deviation is expression of a lesion or compression at the level of the mesencephalic roof.

Vegetative signs

The progressive increase of the arterial systemic pressure with concomitant bradycardia and breathing alterations (Cheines-Stokes respiration) are signs of severe intracranial hypertension with negative prognosis.

The need for a valid system of neurological assessment, highly reproducible, has induced various authors to elaborate systems of evaluation (Plum-Posner, Teasdale-Jennet). Today, the most utilized scale of evaluation is the Glasgow coma scale (GCS) which is based on three parameters: opening of the eyes, verbal response and motor response. Each response is linked to a different score (Table 7.1).

If the summation of the single scores is 7 or less, the patient is in a coma; if the final score is 9 or more, the patient is not in coma. A final score between 13 and 15 corresponds to a patient who is alert or able to wake up.

Although the neurological examination allows a rapid and accurate evaluation of the cerebral conditions of a patient with cranial trauma, some diagnostic radiological procedures, like radiography of the skull, computed tomography (CT), NMR and SPET, can be useful.

When the patient is not in a coma and has a GCS score over 10, radiography of the skull in the three projections (lateral, anteroposterior at 35°, postero-anterior) is sufficient for discovering possible rimae of fractures of the calvaria and cranial basis and fractures of the calvaria with sinking.

When the state of consciousness worsens, signs of neurological deficit or focal or generalized epileptic crises occur, or the GCS score is less than 7-8, it is necessary to perform CT or NMR.

CT allows the visualization of alterations of the soft tissue, osseous fractures (especially depressed fractures), and the presence of foreign bodies or intracranial air.

It is important to identify the location and the nature of space-occupying lesions (hematomas, contusion, edema) and signs of intracranial hypertension.

In the acute stage, the subdural hematoma appears hyperdense for almost 1-3 weeks, followed by an isodense stage (density equal to that of the parenchyma) lasting 10-15 days (during this period there is the risk of overlooking the hematoma). After about 40 days the hematoma appears hypodense.

Contrast medium application is indispensable for identifying a hematoma during the hypodense stage. The contrast medium shows a hyperdense enhancement at the periphery of the hematic collection. The

Tab. 7.1. Glasgow coma scale

Verbal response		Eye-opening response		Motor response	
None	1	None	1	None	1
Incomprehensible sounds	2	To painful stimulus	2	Extends	2
Inappropriate words	3	To speech	3	Flexes	3
Confused response	4	Spontaneous	4	Withdraws	5
Oriented response	5			Localizes	5
				Obeys command	6

epidural hematoma has a typical hyperdense biconvex appearance, like a "biconvex lens".

The subarachnoid hemorrhage is characterized by hyperdense areas which outline the subarachnoid spaces.

The cerebral contusions appear as dyshomogeneous hyper- and hypo-dense areas, in relation to hemorrhagic alterations, edema or tissular necrosis, and are often associated with signs of mass effect.

Angiographical examination is now considered obsolete for the study of intracranial post-traumatic lesions. It can be useful in cases of a hematoma isodense to the cerebral parenchyma (the hematoma appears like an avascular space between brain and cranial theca) or in cases of coma depassè where the absence of filling of the intracranial tract of the carotid artery is a sign of cerebral death.

Cerebral NMR has a lower diagnostic value compared to CT for the diagnosis of traumatic lesions in an acute stage, mainly because the interpretation of the images is more difficult. On the contrary, it is very useful for the interpretation of the traumatic outcomes at the level of the cerebral parenchyma.

SPET allows monitoring of the cerebral metabolism in the areas damaged by trauma.

Therapy

The best choice of treatment in a patient with cranio-encephalic trauma results from a careful clinical, neurological, and radiological examination in order to establish the type and grade of cerebral damage and the presence of lesions in other organs.

The initial treatment should assure good oxygenation of the blood (to allow normocapnia and normoxia), by maintaining the patency of the airways and assure a sufficient tidal volume by assisted respiration.

The maintenance of normal arterial pressure, generally altered toward hypotension due to traumatic shock or hemorrhagic hypovolemia, is achieved with the restoration of a normal volemia. In cases of hypertension, linked to adrenergic activity, this is achieved with hypotensive drugs or diuretics. Correction of the systemic acidosis (metabolic and respiratory) responsible for hypotension, hypocapnia and apnea, is obtained with endovenous infusion of sodium bicarbonate, while altered hydroelectrolytic equilibrium is restored with infusion of balanced saline solutions.

The increased intracranial pressure due to diffuse cerebral edema can be corrected: by raising the head from the horizontal plane to facilitate venous draining of the intracranial circle at the neck and right atrium; with endovenous administration of hypertonic solutions (osmotic diuretic, mannitol 0.5-1 g/kg) or oral administration of glycerol in association with loop diuretics (furosemide); with high dosages of steroids; with hyperventilation which produces hypocapnia at a pCO_2 of 20-30 mmHg and then vasoconstriction and decrease of the cerebral blood flow and cerebral volume; or with barbiturics (pentobarbital 3-5 mg/kg in one dose followed by continuous infusion of 100-200 mg/h) which decreases by 50% the metabolism and blood cerebral outflow.

In past years, knowledge of biochemical alterations of neuronal cell metabolism caused by cranial trauma (accumulation of intracellular Ca^{+2}, and release of type A free fatty acids, arachidonic acid and oxygen free radicals) has lead to the utilization of drugs which decreasing or block the death of neurons.

Calcium antagonist drugs are used to restore the equilibrium of the intracellular Ca^{2+} (nimodipin, nicardipin). Free-radical scavengers, which act by an antioxidant mechanism (alfatocopherol or vitamin E, ascorbic acid, barbiturics, mannitol), are used to decrease the negative effects on the neuron caused by free fatty acids.

Surgical therapy

This is indicated in all cases where cerebral CT and NMR show lesions responsible for compression and displacement of the cerebral structures.

The traumatic pathologies which require the surgical treatment are: extradural hematomas, subdural hematomas, intracerebral hematomas, lacero-bruising foci with dimensions of over 3 cm and with important mass effect and generalized cerebral edema not sensitive to medical therapy, and depressed fractures of the calvaria with dural laceration. In cases of hematomas and lacero-bruising foci, the operation consists in a craniotomy at the level of the hematic collection, removal of the blood and coagulation of lacerated and bleeding vessels.

In the chronic subdural hematoma, it is sufficient to empty the hematoma by osseous drilling and to open the dura mater and capsule surrounding the lesion.

The prognosis in patients operated for hematoma is more promising the more precocious is the surgical operation.

In open traumas, the immediate surgical operation is necessary to avoid complications, mainly of septic nature (meningitides, encephalitides, abscesses, thrombophlebitis).

The operation consists in the removal of foreign bodies and areas of cerebral parenchymal necrosis, disinfecting the operative hollow and repairing the various anatomical planes turning to, if necessary, skin, osseous and dural plastic.

In patients with intracranial hypertension by diffuse cerebral edema, not sensitive to medical therapy (pressure values, measured and registered with intraventricular cannulas and/or tubes localized in the subdural or extradural spaces, over 50-60 mmHg), the osseous temporal or bilateral frontal or bihemispheric decompression is performed.

8. Functional neurosurgery

Trigeminal neuralgia

Trigeminal neuralgia, also known as painful tic, is a repetitive and unilateral facial pain and is due to various causes. It most frequently involves the right side and affects, mainly adult women in the sixth-seventh decades of life. Trigeminal neuralgia can be caused by several diseases affecting the homolateral trigeminal system. In most cases this neuralgia is essential and seems to be caused by a compression of the trigeminal nerve, at its exit from the pons, by an artery or a tortuous vein nearby. In 5%-8% of cases, the pain is caused by a ponto-cerebellar angle tumor, such as the neurinoma, the meningioma or the epidermoid. In 2%-3% of cases, the pain is caused by multiple sclerosis. Many theories have been formulated to explain the onset of the painful crisis. For example, some believe that demyelinization, due to nerve compression caused by a tumor or a vessel (neurovascular conflict) or due to multiple sclerosis, allows the transmission between close axons. Even if this hypothesis is suggestive, it does not explain why there are long periods of pain remission during the disease evolution.

Symptomatology and diagnosis

The pain begins suddenly, and it is violent and lasts less than one minute. It is spontaneous, however it can be caused by harmless, painless stimuli, such as mastication, speaking, or simply touching part of the facial skin. The pain is unforeseeable, lancinating, like an electrical discharge, localized in a territory innervated by a trigeminal branch. It is similar to the sensation felt when a dentist touches nonanesthetized tooth pulp with a drill. The patient, in fact, initially goes to the dentist who sometimes removes one or more teeth without achieving an improvement of the painful condition.

The neurological examination of essential trigeminal neuralgia is usually negative. If the neuralgia is due to multiple sclerosis or to a ponto-cerebellar angle tumor, trigeminal hypoesthesia is found, often associated with other cranial nerve or long pyramidal tract deficits. The clinical diagnosis is confirmed by cerebral CT or NMR, which can exclude the presence of expansive lesions.

There are numerous therapeutic possibilities and none is superior to the others. Usually, the patient with painful tic undergoes more than one therapeutic treatment during disease evolution. It is evident that, if the neuralgia is caused by a tumor compressing the nerve, the tumor must be removed with a surgical operation.

Medical therapy

There are some antiepileptic drugs which seem to decrease the painful tic. Carbamazepine is initially administered at doses of 400 mg/day and it is progressively decreased until reaching the lower dose which can avoid the pain onset. High doses can be badly tolerated and they can cause drowsiness. This drug can also cause leukopenia and it can modify the hepatic functions. Other used drugs are fenitoine, initially administrated at a dose of 100 mg (three times a day) and baclofen (5-10 mg, three times a day). These drugs become inefficacious in time and the patient must increase the dose, causing the onset of side effects. Sometimes it is necessary to switch from one drug to another or to associate more drugs.

Surgical therapy

Injection or avulsion of the peripheral branches

One of the branches of the trigeminal nerve can be either infiltrated with neurolytic substances, such as alcohol, or it can be surgically cut. After the infiltration, an anesthetized area appears, but in time the nerve regenerates and both sensitivity and pain return. For example, pain can regress for about one year after a supraorbital branch infiltration. Nerve avulsion, instead, causes regression of pain for about 2-3 years.

Trigeminal or gasserian rhizolysis

It is thought that with these procedures, the damage to the ganglion and the sensitive trigeminal nerve roots gives a more lasting analgesia, since the regeneration of these structures occurs more slowly than that of the peripheral branches. In the past, anterior trigeminal rhizotomy was performed by exposing and dividing, partially or totally, the sensitive trigeminal roots close to the gasserian ganglion. Today, this is achieved by inserting a needle in the oval foramen and pushing it into the ganglion, in contact with the sensitive roots. The nervous fiber destruction is achieved either with an injection of neurolytic substances such as glycerol, with radiofrequencies which cause thermic lesions (Fig. 8.1), or by compression of the ganglion with a small balloon joined to a Fogarty catheter (Figs. 8.2; 8.3). With these procedures, the patient does not feel pain for a long time, but a more or less marked area of hypoesthesia is present. The best results are achieved by thermocoagulation: only 25% of patients have a pain relapse within 5 years. Less brilliant results are achieved with glycerolysis, but the most frequent complications of the previous procedure are avoided. These complications are analgesia algera or paralytic keratitis, in case the first branch is involved.

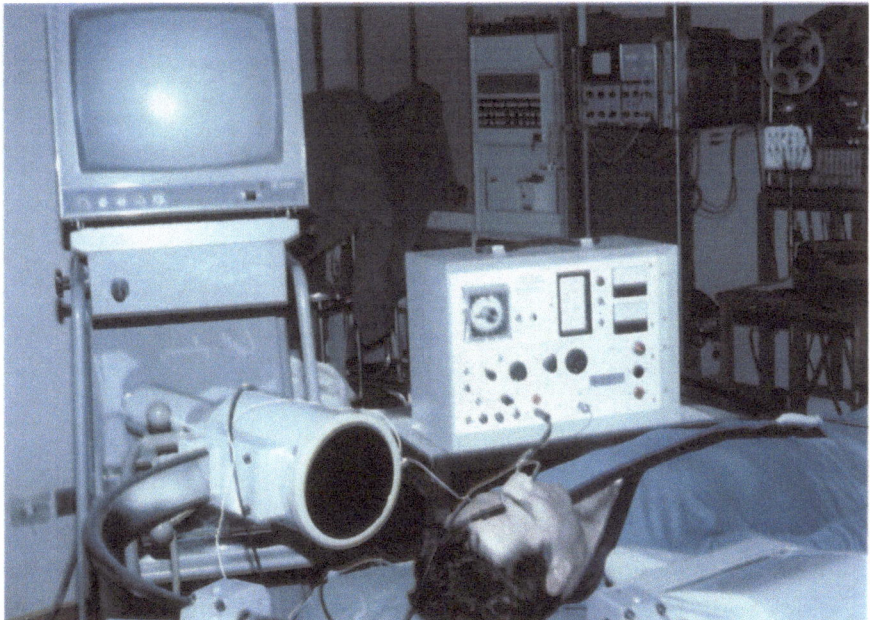

Fig. 8.1. Electrostimulator for thermocoagulation

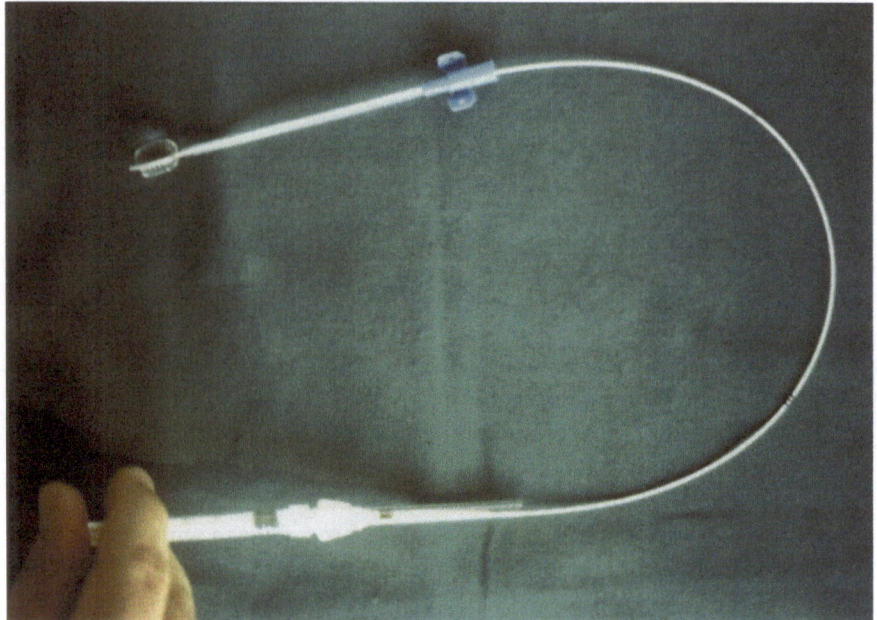

Fig. 8.2. Fogarty catheter with balloon

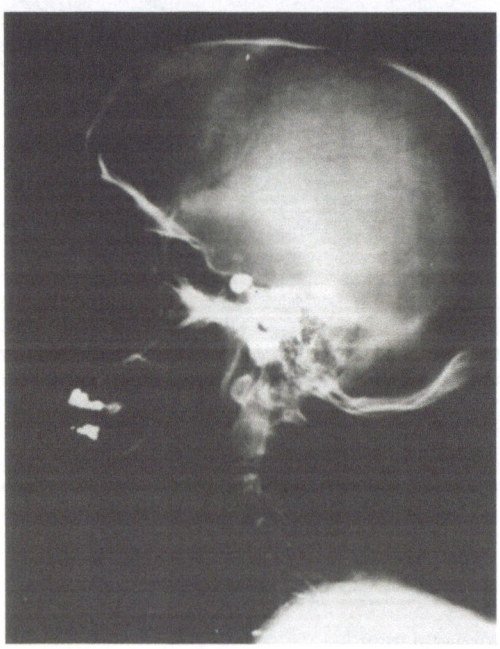

Fig. 8.3. Skull X-ray showing the Fogarty balloon compressing the gasserian ganglion

Microvascular decompression

It is thought that neuralgia is due to trigeminal nerve compression caused by the superior cerebellar artery at the nerve exit from the pons. A suitable microsurgical operation, aiming to a definitive separation between the nerve and the vessel, has been devised: the neurovascular conflict area is reached through a retromastoid suboccipital craniotomy; after separating the nerve from the vessel, an insulating material is inserted between the two structures. In this way, regression of painful symptomatology is achieved, without any disorder to facial sensitivity. The sensitive trigeminal root can be identified and cut in the area close to the pons, if during the operation no conflict is found. In this case, the pain disappears but there is facial hypoesthesia. Finally, it can be said that none of the above procedures is superior to the others for the treatment of trigeminal neuralgia. Each technique has advantages and disadvantages and has to be chosen according to the clinical case. During the disease evolution, each patient usually undergoes more than one of the described procedures to relieve the pain.

Glossopharyngeal neuralgia

It is an infrequent disorder, in fact the ratio between glossopharyngeal (GN) and trigeminal neuralgia (TN) is 1:100. In most cases, this condition affects adults of both sexes and it is often localized on the left side. The pain arises and spreads to any point of the territory innervated by glossopharyngeal fibers. It usually affects the posterior part of the pharynx, the tonsillar region, and the tongue base, and it can irradiate to the ear. In this last case, the pain seems to arise from inside the acoustic canal, at the tympanic region or eustachian canal.

This pain is similar to an electric discharge or stab blow in the throat. It can also be a bothersome sensation, like having a foreign body in the pharynx or ear. This pain is unilateral and intermittent, and it is induced by swallowing and by food-induced salivation. In rare cases, the painful symptomatology can be associated with a syncopal episode of loss of consciousness, characterized by an asystolia which can last more than 30 seconds, such to require a pace-maker installation. The physiological mechanism of this rare phenomenon is unknown, even if diffusion of afferent impulses to the vagal nerve nucleus across the solitary tract and hypersensitivity of the nerve itself have been postulated.

The diagnosis of glossopharyngeal neuralgia is established according to the clinical history, through an accurate examination of the pain characteristics, and head and neck CT and NMR, aiming to exclude the presence of organic lesions. In some cases, the diagnosis can be confirmed by the application of a local anesthetic on the pharyngeal region. In such cases, for about two hours, the painful attacks regress and the patient can eat regularly.

As for the trigeminal neuralgia, the therapy of this disease can be medical or surgical. The medical treatment consists in giving the same drugs used for the painful tic; the surgical treatment consists either in thermocoagulation of cranial nerves IX and X at the jugular foramen, or retromastoid suboccipital craniotomy allowing direct intervention in the posterior cranial fossa. If there is a neurovascular conflict, it is sufficient to separate the nerves from the vessels with insulating material. If there are no anatomical anomalies, it is necessary to perform the complete resection of cranical nerve IX and partial resection of cranical nerve X.

Facial spasm

Facial spasm is a syndrome with gradual onset, characterized by intermittent contraction of the muscles responsible for facial mimicry. The typical clinical picture is characterized by a contraction beginning at eye level, then spreading to the other hemifacial muscles, platysma included. In other cases, the facial spasm can begin at the muscles of the mouth.

Usually, a series of jerks is observed, not associated with lacrimation, which become increasingly frequent and intense and are followed by a continuous muscle contraction, lasting up to one minute. They can be induced by voluntary muscle movements and increase with fatigue, anxiety and stress. Head and body movements can also modify the intensity of the spasms, which can occur even while sleeping.

This disease mainly affects adult women. At first, it mainly represents an esthetic problem but, when the attacks become more frequent and intense, the binocular vision can be affected compromising other activities such as reading or driving a car.

The diagnosis is mainly achieved by clinical observation. However, tests such as CT and NMR are necessary to exclude other pathological processes in the posterior cranial fossa, such as vascular malformations of the posterior circle (dolichomegabasilar, aneurysms, angiomas, tumors). Even if the facial spasm is due to a neurovascular conflict, the neuroradiologic tests does not always show a vascular anomaly.

This syndrome can sometimes be associated with a dysfunction in the homolateral acoustic and trigeminal nerves. In these cases, the patient reports tinnitus, hypoacusis and vestibular disorders. Furthermore, it is not rare to observe essential arterial hypertension. This hypertension regresses or improves after a surgical operation in the posterior cranial fossa. Some authors think that this is due to the same vascular anomaly causing a compression at the level of the bulbar olive. The hypertension has been noticed when the left bulbar olive was involved. A condition of neurovascular conflict is one of the factors causing the syndrome. In most cases this is caused by the posterior-inferior (PICA) or the anterior-inferior cerebellar artery (AICA). In particular, it has been postulated that the nerve is affected in a crucial point corresponding to the junction between the glial and non-glial parts. Anatomical studies revealed that the distance between this point, without myelinic insulation, and brainstem is of about 2.5 cm.

Several kinds of invasive and noninvasive therapies have been used, but with scarce results. Carbamazepine, baclofen, botulin toxin, psychotherapy, electric stimulations and radiotherapy by linear accelerator are some of the noninvasive therapies used. The interruption of the peripheral branches of the facial nerve, the nerve section at the level of the stylomastoid foramen and the consecutive anastomosis with the hypoglossal nerve, the nerve decompression inside the facial canal, and the resolution of the neurovascular conflict at the ponto-cerebellar angle are among the surgical techniques used (Figs. 8.4; 8.5). All these procedures share the disadvantage of being followed, sooner or later, by the reappearance of the disorders. Recently, small doses of botulin exotoxin were introduced inside the muscles innervated by the facial nerve, obtaining the disappearance of the disorders in almost all cases, but with temporany effects. However, this technique can be repeated with no disadvantages.

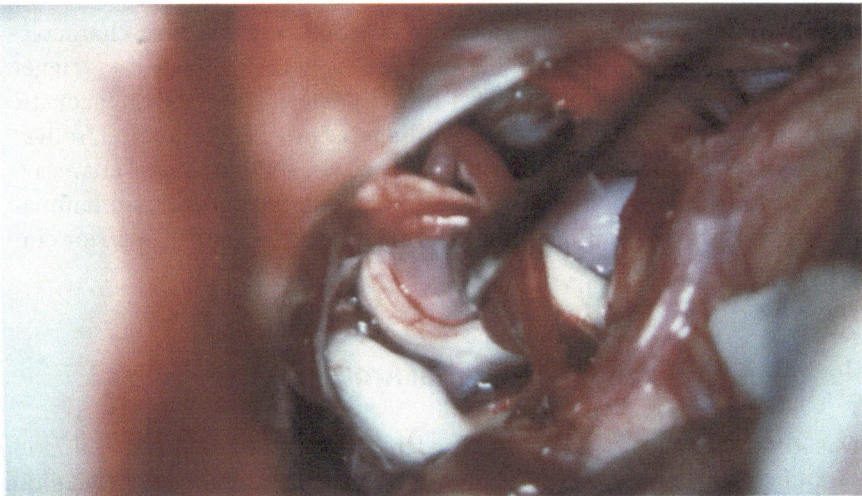

Fig. 8.4. Surgical aspect of neurovascular conflict between cranial nerve VII and AICA

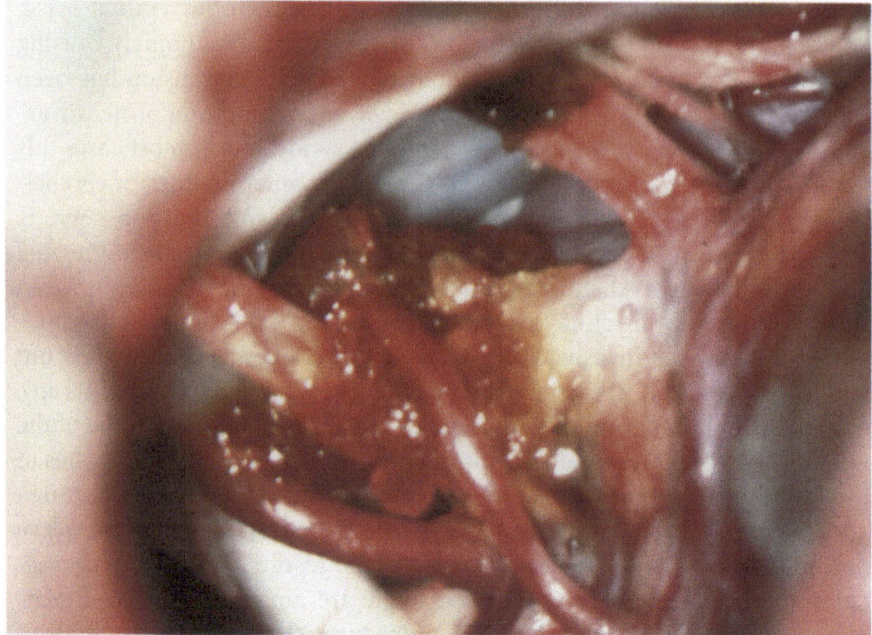

Fig. 8.5. Surgical aspect after muscle interposition between cranial nerve VII and AICA

Neuralgia of the intermediate nerves

It is a painful syndrome, with unknown etiology. It is very rare, characterized by brief but intense painful crises felt deeply inside the ear. A "trigger area" is usually present at the level of the posterior part of the acoustic canal. The pain can be associated with alterations of lacrimation, salivation and taste. The association with herpes zoster is frequent (Ramsay-Hunt's syndrome). The therapy is based on analgesic and anti-inflammatory drugs or on sectioning of the intermediate nerve in the posterior cranial fossa.

Neuralgia of the greater occipital Arnold's nerve

The symptomatology is characterized by paroxysmal, monolateral, and painful crises (like the thrust of a knife), starting from the superior region of the neck, with irradiation to the occipital region and vertix, and to the posterior parietal and retromastoid regions. The crises are often induced by the simple skiming of the scalp in the occipital region, by flexion and rotation movements of the neck and by compression of the nerve emergence point (2-3 cm laterally to the external occipital protuberance). The neurological examination and neuroradiological tests are negative. The therapy consists in the nerve blockage by local anesthetics or in alcoholization.

Secondary occipital neuralgia

It is a prolonged contracture of the occipitonuchal and neck muscles caused by arthrosis, forced position of the head, rheumatic myositis and anxiety neurosis. The pain is bilateral, not very intense, without a precise localization, with an insidious onset, and often associated with stiffness of the neck muscles. The therapy is based on antidepressant and anti-inflammatory drugs.

Great auricular nerve neuralgia

This is a rare, painful syndrome, characterized by auricular painful crises, induced by contact at the level of the auricle. The pain can be associated with vegetative phenomena and has a weekly frequency, higher during winter months. The therapy consists in the administration of anti-inflammatory drugs.

Charlin's syndrome

It is a complex syndrome characterized by nasal paroxysmal pains, and nasal and ocular disorders. This syndrome seems to be related to irritative phenomena of the nasociliar nerve and its terminal branches, due to direct factors (sinusitis, traumatic or neoplastic lesions) or reflex stimuli (nasal deviation) determining a vascular mechanism of the neurovegetative type. Pain is violent, burning, and can last from a few minutes to a few hours, with localization in the lateral wall of the nasal fossa and irradiation to the orbital cavity, nose wing and frontal region. The therapy consists in local anesthesia or in the use of topical vasoconstrictors.

Sluder's syndrome

This syndrome seems to be related to an irritative and idiopathic stress of the sphenopalatine ganglion. Sometimes it can be due to sphenoid or ethmoid sinusitis, or to traumatic or neoplastic lesions of the pterigomaxillary fossa. The pain arises from the deep part of a nasal fossa and of the rhinopharyngeal cavity, with possible irradiation to the orbit cavity, palate, mastoid occiput and nucha. Rhinorrhea and/or nasal obstruction, scialorrhea, lacrimation, ocular mucosal congestion, photophobia and disorders of taste perception at the level of the anterior two-thirds the tongue are associated symptoms. The treatment consists in anesthetizing the sphenopalatine ganglion by anesthesia on the nasal mucosa of the medium turbinate.

Chronic pain

Pain is often the first symptom and common denominator of several diseases, such as headache in cerebral tumors, angina in coronary diseases, and post-prandial weight in the upper right quadrant of the abdomen in cholecystitis. Therefore, pain can be considered a defense of the body, although debilitating. From an *etiological* point of view, there are two types of pain: *benign* and *malignant*. Benign pain is due to several causes; malignant pain is often associated with neoplasias.

From a *physiological* point of view, pain can be divided into: *somatic* (due to tissural damage and the release of neurohumoral substances), and *neurogenic* or by *deafferentation* (due to a lesion of the central or peripheral nervous system).

From a *temporal* point of view pain can be acute, if it has occurred for a short time and disappears promptly, or chronic, if it is persistent and disappears with difficulty.,

Neuroanatomy and neurophysiology of pain

It is necessary to know the anatomy and physiology of pain in order to understand its causes and find the treatments to relieve it. The peripheral nerves transmit important sensory information from the body to the various nerve centers: spinal cord, brainstem and cerebral cortex.

The skin, mucous membranes and periost can be considered the most peripheral parts of the nervous system because these structures contain sensory receptors. The nerve-free endings are pain receptors; the nervous impulses generated by these endings are conducted to "central centers" by the peripheral nerves. Two subtypes of these peripheral fibers transmit the pain sensation: the C non-myelinated fibers conduct an aching, indeterminated pain sensation and the delta-A myelinated fibers conduct an acute and localized pain.

The cell bodies of the afferent nociceptive fibers are localized in the dorsal ganglions of the nerve roots and in the gasserian ganglion of the trigeminal roots. These neurons are bipolar and connected (centrally) to the spinal cord or the brainstem. The central fibers of the primary nociceptive afferences (delta A and C fibers) terminate in the superficial layer of the dorsal spinal cord, specifically at the level of the I, II, III Rexed's laminae. The primary integration of the painful information occurs in this region, called "dorsal root entry zone" (DREZ).

The fibers of the neurons localized in the DREZ (secondary nociceptive afferences) project to the thalamus and form the spinothalamic tract. This tract decussates at the midline and crosses the spinal cord anterolateral column. There are additional secondary afferences sending information directly to the brainstem reticular substance. Both the direct spinothalamic tract and the spinoreticulothalamic tract reach the centrobasal complex of the thalamus. From the thalamus, tertiary fibers depart and project to the primary and secondary somatosensory areas of the cerebral cortex.

There is an additional neural system for pain control. The alpha-A and beta-A big myelinated fibers of the peripheral nerves inhibit spinothalamic neurons. This effect is probably due to inhibitory interneurons, localized at all levels of the II and III laminae of the dorsal horns. Furthermore, neurons localized in the posterior horns can inhibit thalamic nociceptive cells.

Neurosurgical treatments

Peripheral procedures

Several surgical techniques can relieve pain. The section of the peripheral nerve (peripheral neurectomy) can abolish the pain, but this approach causes several problems. First, pain is rarely perceived in a region innervated by a single nerve fiber due to the overlapping peripheral nerve distribution. Second, peripheral neurectomy often causes serious neurological deficits because most peripheral nerves are both sensory and motor. This technique is rarely used, with the exception of the treatment of pain due to superficial radial nerve lesions. Peripheral nerve stimulation is used to relieve chronic pain due to nervous lesions. With this technique, by transcutaneous implantation, the myelinated fibers inhibiting the nociceptive fibers at the level of the posterior horns are stimulated.

Rhizotomy consists in sectioning the sensitive fibers of the nerve roots. This technique can be extradural or intradural. In the first case, the whole posterior root is sectioned, in the second case only part of the radicles is sectioned. The ventrolateral part of the nervous radicles is dissected with the *selective posterior rhizotomy*. Rhizotomy is utilized when the pain is induced by brachial plexus tumors (Pancoast's syndrome), thoracic cage tumors, or pelvis tumors. It is rarely utilized for the treatment of benign lesion because it can induce a painful syndrome by deaffferentation (post-rhizotomy dysesthesia).

The removal of the sensory ganglion (*gangliotomy*) is recommended for the treatment of localized malignant pain. The gangliotomy is preferable to the posterior rhizotomy because 20% of the afferent nociceptive fibers is associated with the ventral roots.

Central procedures

Spinal cord

Several procedures to relieve chronic pain are performed at spinal cord level. The aim of these techniques is the section of the ventral spinothalamic tract (cordotomy) by laminectomy or by a percutaneous approach using radiofrequency electrodes. Cordotomy causes a contralateral analgesia below the lesion and relieves the malignant pain, which is mainly unilateral. The post-cordotomy dysesthesia (due to deafferentation) limits the use of cordotomy to malignant lesions.

Stimulation of the spinal cord dorsal columns (*spinal stimulators)* has been used for benign chronic pain, especially lumbar pain due to discopathy. The spinal stimulators relieve the pain by stimulating the descending inhibitory contingent. During the stimulation, paresthesias are perceived with the same distribution of the pain.

Intraspinal narcotic analgesia is based on the instillation of small doses of morphine directly into the cerebrospinal fluid or in the epidural space, inducing a prolonged and deep analgesia in case of metastatic malignant pains.

Brain

Procedures of stimulation or ablation are used on the brain as in the spinal cord. Stereotactic techniques are utilized in mesencephalic and diencephalic regions. *Stereotactic mesencephalotomy* is used for cervicobrachial neoplastic pain or for thalamic pain. Brainstem or thalamic stimulation (*deep cerebral stimulation*) has been used in both malignant and benign pains. The analgesia caused by brainstem stimulation seems to be due to opioid substances, unlike thalamic stimulation.

The hypophysectomy is a good central procedure for the treatment of pain caused by osseous metastases. The pituitary gland can be removed by transphenoidal approach or it can be destroyed by alcohol. The`pain disappears especially in hormone-dependent tumors (prostate, breast).

Deafferentation pain

Deafferentation gives a particularly painful sensation (burning, lancinating, pulsating) in a body region which is partially or totally insensitive because the peripheral nociceptive receptors are disconnected from central structures.

Several deafferentation painful syndromes occur after limb amputation (50%-90%), root avulsion (80%-90%) and peripheral nerve trauma, and in paraplegia, tetraplegia (10%-20%), and post-herpetic neuralgia. The causes of this type of pain are unknown. It has been suggested that deafferentation causes spinal neuronal hyperactivity, which is perceived as a painful sensation. This neurophysiological hyperactivity may be due to a hypersensitivity of the disconnected central neurons (as an epileptogenic focus), to a lack of influence of the central inhibitory system, or to a modification of the local concentration of neurotransmitters.

Studies of the anatomy and physiology of the spinal cord posterior horns has led Nashold to think that these regions, responsible for pain transmission, are "non-functional" rather than "diseased". For this reason he operated on the DREZ causing lesions in the entry zone of the nerve roots according to the pain location. The aim of this procedure is to convert an injured region (in theory, hyperactive) into a quiescent scar. Small electrodes are placed in the spinal cord to induce injuries by radiofrequency at different levels. This procedure on the DREZ was initially performed on patients with pain due to brachial plexus avulsion, achieving pain disappearance in 66% of cases.

Since then, this technique has been employed for the treatment of the previously described painful syndromes. Recently, it has been used in post-thoracotomy cases or in post-herpetic ophthalmic neuralgia. In the latter case, the injury is made on the DREZ of the trigeminal inferior nucleus.

Further intracranial procedures

Several cerebral structures can be operated on, using stereotactic surgery, to achieve pain remission. These structures are usually localized in the thalamus: dorsal medial (DM), ventral posterolateral (VPL), central medial (CM) nuclei and the pulvinar. The periaqueductal mesencephalic region (PMR) and the spinothalamic lemniscus in the pons are also included.

The effects of thalamic nuclei electrical stimulation on pain were studied in 1950. Reynolds (1969) studied the stimulus-induced analgesia (SIA) caused by electrical stimulation of the PMR. Subsequent studies ascribed the SIA efficacy to endogenous opioid substances production by the PMR, with activation of the pain inhibitory descendent system extending from the PMR to the spinal cord posterior horns. Pain inhibition occurs with a serotonin-mediated mechanism and, probably, with other neuropeptides.

In order to have a successful procedure, it is necessary to carry out a careful selection of patients. First of all, the pain must be very intense, persisting for at least 6-12 months, and being such that the patient cannot lead a normal life. The pain must be drug-resistant or insensitive to therapies such as transcutaneous electrical stimulation, acupuncture and nerve blockage. It is also important to understand the patient's psychology.

The surgical procedure is carried out with local anesthesia and under slight sedation. A stereotactic helmet is applied with the base parallel to the orbito-meatal line and a precoronal hole is drilled two centimeters from the midline. At this point, there are a few possibilities: we can affect a recording, a stimulation or a coagulation of the selected target after its identification. For example, low frequency periventricular stimulation of the griseum causes diplopia, anxiety, and sensation of heat. Higher frequency stimulation causes eye deviation, upward gaze limitation, heart rate and arterial pressure increase. The activity of the ventral posterior nucleus cells can be recorded at rest or after activation by contralateral cutaneous tactile stimulation.

After the selected target is identified, we must decide if it will be chronically stimulated or it will be destroyed. In the first case, the patient is exposed to electrical stimulation for some days to verify if the painful symptomatology disappears. If so, a permanent device is applied. In the second case, thalamotomy is performed by electrocoagulation.

9. Spinal dysraphias

Spina bifida

This myelovertebral malformation can be distinguished into two forms: occult spina bifida and cystic spina bifida.

Occult spina bifida

It is characterized by the lack of closure of the posterior vertebral arches, usually at lumbar or sacral level, rarely at cervical level. It can involve the dura mater and the spinal cord. Fibrous or adipose tissue is interposed between the two stump extremities of the arch, resembling a tumor. The fibroadipose mass can compress or penetrate the dural sac and involve the roots. In light forms, it can be asymptomatic and only an hypertrichosis area above the schisis can be observed. Radiography (Fig. 9.1) and CT show absence of part of the posterior arch. When there is an involvement of the dura or of the roots, we can observe dorsolumbar pain, accentuation of the lumbar lordosis and deep hyporeflexia; if the sacral roots are severely involved, we can observe "saddle" hypo-anesthesia and sphincteric disorders. Myelo-CT shows a hyperdense area in the spinal canal and/or in the spinal sac. NMR perfectly shows the modifications of the soft tissues, such as lipoma (hyperintense on T2-weighted images), or the anatomical modifications of the nervous structures often associated with this pathology (terminal filum anchorage, myelomeningocele, Arnold-Chiari malformation, syringomyelia).

Therapy. Operation, by microsurgical technique, allows an almost complete separation of the lipomatous mass from the roots and/or from the cone.

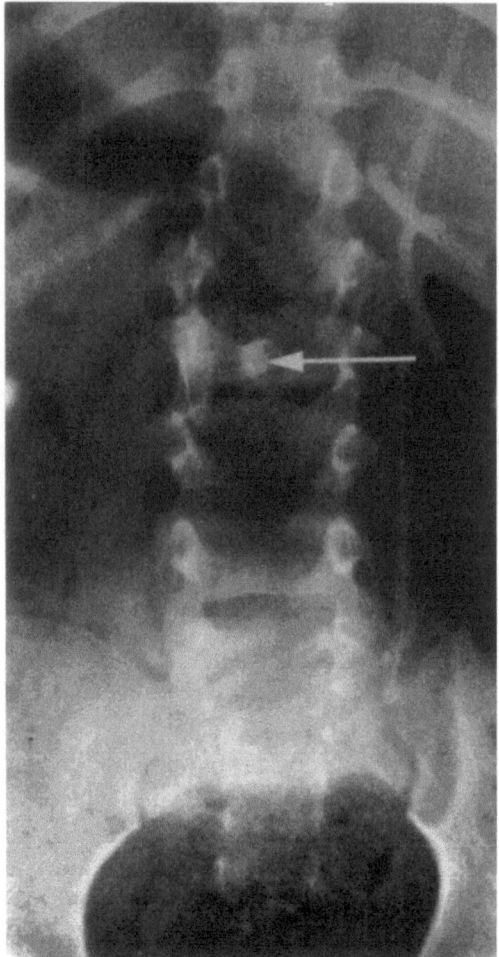

Fig. 9.1. Lumbo-sacral X-ray: occult spina bifida with osseous beak

Cystic spina bifida

It is a myelodysplasia with rachischisis and it can be present in three forms listed below.

Myelocele or myeloschisis

It is the most severe form, usually extending to most all of the spinal cord, which is often rudimentary and covered by the arachnoid only due to the absence of the meninges and vertebral arches in the posterior part. Due to its severity, it is generally incompatible with life.

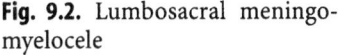

Fig. 9.2. Lumbosacral meningo-
myelocele

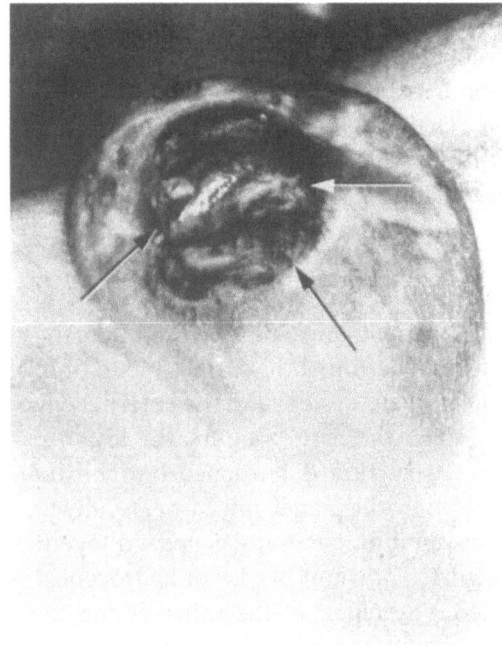

Myelomeningocele

It is a dorsolumbar median sac, above the vertebral schisis, filled with cerebrospinal fluid. It contains nerve roots and portions of spinal cord (Fig. 9.2).

To the external inspection, the sac is formed by a central area called medullary sac or neural plate, formed by spinal cord and surrounded by a epitheliomeningeal area (thickned arachnoid) and by a dermic area formed by either normal or atrophic skin. In some cases, there is no sac but a lipomatous mass covered with normal skin, adhering to the roots and the spinal cord, herniating through a schisis. Hydrocephalus can be found in 80% of patients affected by myelomeningocele. Agenesis of the corpus callosum, Arnold-Chiari malformation, transparent septum cyst, or a midline lipoma can be present.

In these malformations the motor deficits consist in flaccid paralysis with sphincteric disorders. If the localization is at S1-S2 level, only the feet are paralyzed; if at S3-S5 level there are only sphincteric disorders. It should be underlined that motility worsens rapidly after birth, even within a few hours or days. Sensory deficiences with analogous distribution are also associated.

Plain film and CT show the osseous malformations related to this pathology, essentially spina bifida. NMR is the best method to evaluate the malformations of the nervous structures and of the meninges. This test shows the posterior herniation, not covered with cutaneous structures, dural sac and neural elements.

The myelomeningocele can cause serious complications: septic complications (myelitis, meningitis, encephalitis) that are often fatal, hydrocephalus, and trophic disorders (decubitus wounds, perianal and vulvar ulcers).

Therapy

The patient must be operated shortly after birth, preferably within 36 hours. The aim of the surgical operation is to reconstruct a barrier between the nervous system and the external environment.

After the first 36 hours, the lesion is almost surely colonized and the reconstruction is burdened by high mortality and morbidity. In case of infection, the plaque must be carefully washed with sterile solutions. A specific antibiotic therapy is needed together with application of an external ventricular shunt in case of hydrocephalus with cerebrospinal canal infection. The repair of the spinal lesion and the application of a ventricular shunt will be performed only when three consecutive caltures are sterile.

Some newborns are not only affected by spinal malformations and hydrocephalus but also by serious spinal and upper limb deformities with congenital or traumatic abnormalities in other areas. These patients would not get a real benefit from an early surgical operation and a more conservative treatment is appropriate. The surgical operation should be delayed at least for a month, hoping that the patient survives until then.

Meningocele

It is constituted by an arachnoid diverticulum protruding through a schisis, not containing nervous roots or spinal cord. It is similar to a lumbosacral sac, of varying volume, with thick and hypertrichotic or angiomatous skin, and containing cerebrospinal fluid. The sac is connected with the vertebral specus (communicating meningocele) or it can be isolated by arachnoid membranes (excluded meningocele). In some cases, the malformation is associated with myelodysplasia. The best test for the diagnosis of this malformation is NMR, which shows the cystic formation covered with dermic structures containing cerebrospinal fluid without neural elements. Complications are possible if the meningocele is ulcerated.

Therapy

The surgical operation is essential and definitive.

Diastematomyelia

The spinal cord is divided into two halves by an osseous spur which arises from the anterior part of the spinal canal. The diastematomyelia can either involve only one tract of the spinal cord or be extended. Clinically, at the time of the first footsteps, the child shows difficulty in walking and sphincteric incontinence. Sometimes, on the contrary, the symptoms are scarce during the first years of life, occuring later with spastic paraparesis, sensory disorders, sphincteric disturbances, and feet ulcerations.

The rachis radiography shows the osseous spur, sometimes associated with a vertebral schisis. CT clearly shows the osseous spur which divides, wholly or partially, the vertebral canal into two parts, often asymmetric, each containing a dural sac with a hemi-spinal cord. NMR images are also detailed and show the spinal cord divided into two structures by an osseous septum.

Therapy is surgical and consists in the removal of the osseous spur and possible lipomatous masses. After the surgical operation, 45% of patients improve, but for about 50% the situation is unvaried.

Spinal dermic sinus

It is a communication, covered by epithelium, between the cutaneous surface and spinal tissue. It can be found on the midline at any level, from the sacrum to the cervical column. It can terminate in the subcutaneous tissue or reach the deepest layers up to the subdural space. This malformation can be associated with posterior spina bifida. Tumors can be found along its extension. The spinal dermic sinus must be distinguished from sinus pilonidalis, which is present in the intergluteal area associated with acute or chronic infections, but with no osseous defects, and does not reach the spinal canal.

At the sacrococcygeal level, this communication rarely extends into the spinal canal or causes meningitis. It can have cranial or caudal direction, inserting itself into the coccyx extremity. Above this level, this malformation is more frequent and reaches the dural level. It can be covered with hairs and is often unobserved. As the cranial dermic sinus, the spinal dermic sinus can be asymptomatic. In some cases it can cause a meningitis, or it can be associated with a dysembryogenetic tumor or with other anomalies, such as lumbosacral lipoma, lumbar meningocele or diastematomyelia.

The radiological diagnosis is achieved by NMR, myelo-CT, and plain films. The introduction of contrast medium into the dermic sinus, to evaluate its direction and extent, is not advisable.

The surgical operation of the sacrococcygeal dermic sinus is not necessary, because in most cases it is extraspinal. On the contrary, the dermic sinus found at higher levels of the vertebral column must be removed as far as its end, without causing neurological damage.

Tethered cord syndrome

With this words we refer to a low medullary cone, anchored by a short terminal filum, to cicatricial adhesions or an intradural lesion, or to both of them. In some patients we can find cutaneous anomalies (for example, a subcutaneous lipoma penetrating through the muscular levels and adhering to the nervous tissue, or hypertrichosis) or scoliosis.

Most patients present hyposthenia of the lower limbs, associated with hypotrophies, sensitivity disorders and vescical dysfunction. Another common symptom is pain, mainly vertebral, sometimes irradiated to the lower limbs and soles of the feet.

The radiological diagnosis is effected with myelography or NMR: these tests show a medullary shadow, extending towards the sacrum and occasionally associated with a filling deficit, due to a satellite lipoma. At lumbar level, the roots come out from the medullary shadow; if the terminal filum is larger than 2 mm, it is normally a short and thick one.

The surgical operation depends on the complexity of the lesion. When the terminal filum is short, without other anomalies, it is dissected between two clips. On the contrary, the surgical procedure is more difficult in presence of adherences or in case of spinal cord sacralization associated with lipoma. In this case, the adherences must be separated carefully, the filum must be dissected and, if there are no tenacious adherences, the lipoma must be separated from the nervous tissue. The surgical results depend on the precocity of the diagnosis and on the seriousness of the neurological deficits. The spinal curvature also is of notable importance, since in 30% of cases scoliosis becomes of surgical interest.

Lumbosacral lipoma

A subcutaneous lipoma, which is normally found at lumbar level, can extend, through a posterior spina bifida, as far as the subdural compartment, adhering more or less strictly to a low medullary cone, to the cauda equina or to the terminal filum. Sometimes, the subcutaneous lipoma is associated with other forms of occult spinal dysraphism, such as a dermic sinus, diastematomyelia or a thickened filum.

The subcutaneous mass is formed by normal adipous tissue, without a capsule. It extends through the spina bifida as far as the dural sac: the intradural extension can be either a small area of fusion with the nervous tissue or a big mass occupying the whole lumbar and sacral canal. The insertion point of the lipoma on the nervous tissue is formed by a dense layer of connective tissue, penetrating into the depth of the nervous structures. In this case the complete removal of a lipoma can cause damage.

The subcutaneous lipoma is present at birth and it rarely grows with time, unless there is an increase in body fat; it is found on the midline as a compressible, but not as a cystic mass. If the mass is lateral and associated with a cyst, it is probably a meningocele or a myelomeningocele, associated with a lipoma. In the last case, the first lamina above the lipoma can be a fibrous or cartilaginous band, compressing the herniated spinal cord and determining, after birth, a worsening of the neurological deficit. Initially, most patients are asymptomatic, showing the first, modest disorders during childhood (sensory deficit in the sacral territories and vesical disorders).

The radiological diagnosis can be done using plain films, myelo-CT and above all MRI, which shows the lipoma extent and its connections with the nervous system.

The aim of surgical operation is to remove the compression and the traction on the nervous tissue. The lipoma appears as a well-circumscribed mass, which must be followed as far as the vertebral level. The lipoma removal is achieved at the operating microscope with the aid of a Cavitron or Laser. A partial removal is usually preferable than a risky dissection, since the decompression is sufficient to stabilize the clinical picture. A subsequent increase in dimensions of the adipous tissue usually depends on body fat increase.

Syringomyelia

It is an intramedullary cavity primitively localized in the commissura cinerea, with successive invasion of the posterior and anterior horns of the spinal cord. It can have notable dimensions and it can involve many medullary metamers. The most frequent site is the cervical enlargement; this cavity contains sallow fluid. The clinical picture is characterized by suspended thermoalgesia hypo-anesthesia, atrophy of small hand muscles, with subsequent extension to proximal segments of the upper limbs and sympa-

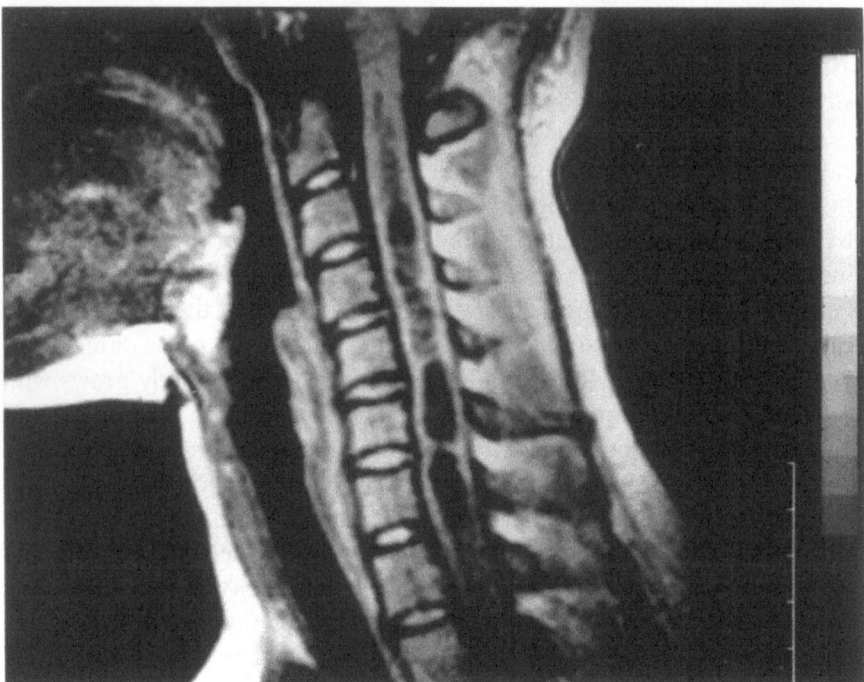

Fig. 9.3. Cervico-dorsal syringomyelia. NMR, T1-weighted image, sagittal view. Presence of voluminous septated syringomyelic cavity localized in the whole cervical spine and upper portion of the dorsal spine

thethic disorders. At an advanced stage, pyramidal and sensory disorders can be present.

CT shows the hypodense area of the intramedullary cyst, but slow myelo-CT is more informative. This test is carried out 8-10 hours after intrathecal introduction of contrast medium which shows the opacification of the cystic cavity, the more intense opacification of the subarachnoid spaces and the medullary thinning surrounding the cyst.

NMR shows the extent of the cavity and its transverse diameter, variable from filiform to massive. It sometimes shows the intracavitary transverse septi and the "glove finger" appearance of the cranial extremity (Figs. 9.3; 9.4).

Therapy. The surgical procedure consists in syringotomy, namely the creation of a connection, after laminectomy, between the cavity and the subarachnoid space with a thin catheter left in situ. Sometimes the operation consists in the application of a shunt between the cavity and the peritoneal space (mainly in hydromyelia cases). Another efficacious therapy for

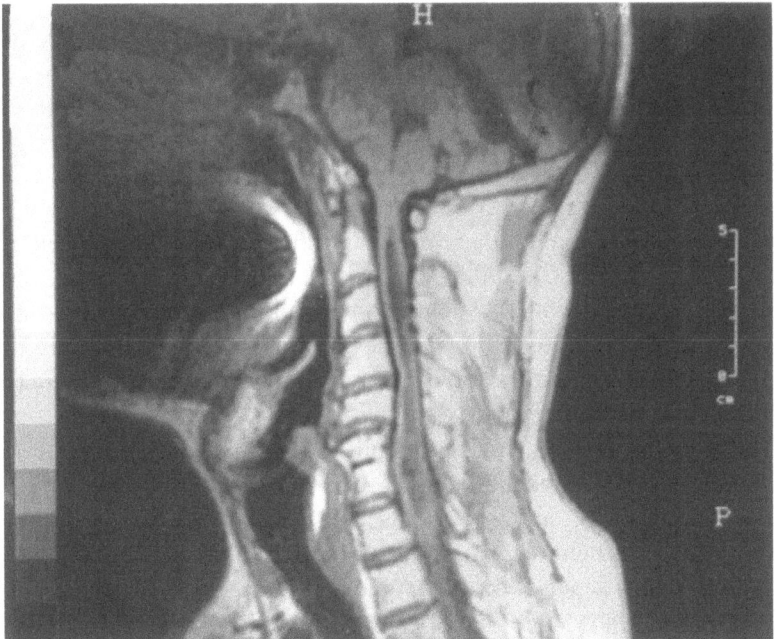

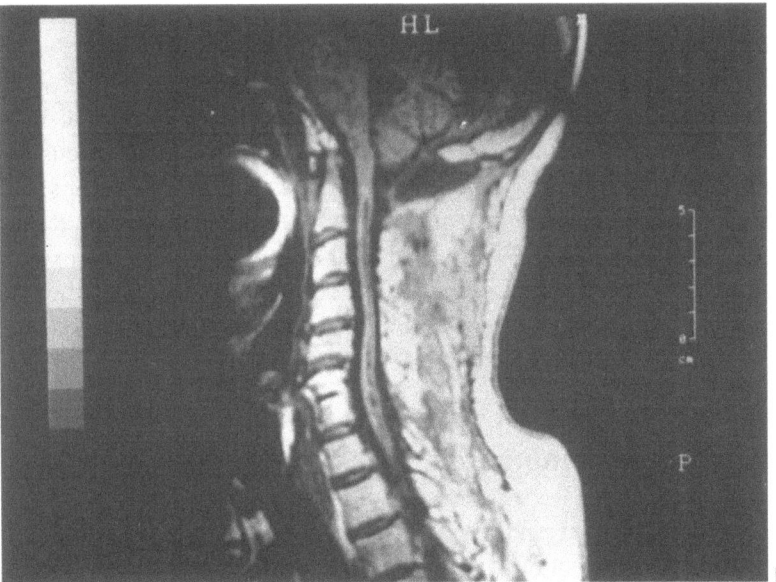

Fig. 9.4a,b. Cervical syringomyelia. NMR, T1-weighted image, sagittal view, before (a) and after (b) surgical treatment. Presence of a syringomyelic cavity with extension from C1 to C7 (a). The post-surgical image shows the decrease of the cavity

syringomyelia is the decompression of the occipital foramen and superior cervical canal, if it is associated with Arnold-Chiari malformation.

Neuroenteric cyst

This cyst can be intramedullary or intradural-extramedullary, localized on the ventral surface of the spinal cord, where it can cause a compression. It derives from endodermic tissue dorsally displaced in the spinal canal, in front of the neural plate. Abnormalities of the vertebral bodies are therefore frequent. A communication can persist (anterior spina bifida) between an intraspinal neuroenteric cyst and a mediastinal cyst.

The cyst contains a colorless fluid, sometimes described as being brownish yellow. The most affected levels are the thoracic, cervical or cervico-thoracic (always above T7). The cysts are covered with a simple or pluristratified epithelium, sometimes associated with a muscular layer. The symptomatology depends on the medullary compression, but clinical pictures with meningitic onset have been observed. Most patients are between 0 and 5 years old. In this case, a paravertebral cyst associated with defects of the vertebral bodies can be frequently observed, even in patients older than 20 years.

An intraspinal neuroenteric cyst is rarer than the cyst of the posterior mediastinum. However, if the mass is localized in the right cervico-thoracic level and vertebral anomalies are associated, an intraspinal extension can be suspected. Therefore, a differential diagnosis with other lesions, such as posterior mediastinum neurogenic tumors, becomes important. Radiological tests such as CT and NMR are crucial as they can show the extent and anatomical connections of the cyst. The surgical treatment of the enterogenic cyst consists in drainage and in a conservative resection of the wall adherent to the spinal cord.

Anterior sacral meningocele

In this rare malformation the spinal sacral meninges are herniated into the pelvis through a defect of the anterior sacral wall, causing local symptoms, due to compression, on the bladder, rectum or other pelvic organs (90% of patients are women).

The sacral defect is variable, sometimes involving the whole coccyx and some sacral segments. The meningocele is full of liquid and it is placed in the retroperitoneal space. The sac, with a wall constituited of arachnoid, dura mater and fibrous tissue, communicates with the sacral subarachnoid space through a tight neck, which penetrates in an ample sacral defect. In rare cases, the sac can herniate through the sciatic foramen and develop in the gluteal region. The cauda equina and the terminal filum are normal, but there are adherences anchoring the nervous structures to the dura mater.

The symptomatology usually occurs around the second or third decade of life and consists in rectal disorders (constipation), vescical disorders (incontinence, retention, enuresis, infections of the urinary tract), or female genital system disorders (dystocia, dysmenorrhea). In some cases, headache during defecation has been reported, probably due to a rapid and transient cerebrospinal fluid passage in the spinal compartment.

The differential diagnosis must be effected for other space-occupying lesions in the small pelvis, such as chordomas, chondromas, teratomas, dermoids and other pelvic tumors. The radiological tests include radiography, CT, NMR, echography, urography and cystography.

The surgical treatment consists in a sacral laminectomy, opening of the dura mater, isolation of the nervous structures and closure of the neck with the fascia. The exclusion of the sac can also occur with an extradural approach, but in no case may it be removed.

Tarlov's cyst

In 1938, after anatomical studies of the terminal filum, Tarlov described some cysts of the sacral or coccygeal posterior roots, developing through the dura mater at the level of the junction between root and ganglion. These cysts are filled with a clear liquid and, initially, they were probably in communication with the subarachnoid spaces.

These cysts often are an occasional finding. They may be responsible for lumbar pain or lombosciatalgia. Myelography shows a slow filling of the cysts, generally multiple and in an eccentric position.

Extradural spinal cysts

These cysts are usually found in the thoracic region, but they can involve the cervical or lumbar regions as well. Thoracic cysts usually develop in young patients, and because of the reduced diameter of the dorsal canal, they cause symptoms very early. These cysts adhere to the dura mater with a tight peduncle situated on the median or paramedian side of the posterior surface. They can communicate with the subarachnoid space. Microscopically, they are covered with a layer of arachnoid cells and their wall is formed by connective tissue. The symptomatology is associated with compression of the spinal cord or the nervous roots. The surgical operation consists in the removal of the cyst and closure of the dural defect.

Caudal regression syndrome (sacral agenesis)

It is the consequence of the failed formation of all or some coccygeal, sacral and, sometimes, lumbar vertebral units, together with the corresponding nervous structures. This malformation is rare and can be classified either as sacral agenesis (total or subtotal) or as hemisacrum (when only segments on one side are present). The medullary chord and the dural sac terminate at the level of the normal vertebra. The muscles of the affected areas are immature and badly shaped with an ample zone of fat and few muscular fibers. In the absence of the bone, the space between skin and peritoneum is filled with fat and fibrous connective tissue. 10% of patients affected by sacral agenesis have, at birth, an imperforate anus.

The symptomatology generally occurs around the third-fifth years of life, with the child not being able to control the sphincters: constipation, urinary incontinence, and recurrent infections of the urinary tract are the most common disorders, while gait can be normal if the lumbar vertebrae are not involved. In severe cases, we can observe serious neurological deficits with paralysis, atrophies of the lower limbs and extensive orthopedic deformities with thoracopelvic dysproportion, lumbar kiphosis and equinovarus deformity.

The radiological diagnosis is achieved with plain films, myelography, and NMR. Surgical operation is necessary only in cases where there is an associated occult spinal dysraphism, such as a lumbosacral lipoma.

Sacrococcygeal teratoma

It is a rare childhood tumor, occuring in 1 of in 40 000 births. It mainly affects females and it probably derives from the totipotential cells of the primitive Hensen's node. Most of these tumors are present at birth. They extend toward the sacrum and coccyx, affecting one or both glutei. They can be solid or cystic and develop in the pelvic cavity with various modalities.

These teratomas are asymptomatic masses, but during delivery they can break and bleed. In some cases, obstructive symptoms of the urinary or digestive system can occur. The sacrococcygeal teratoma must be distinguished from the lipoma, the myelomeningocele, the retrorectal abscess and other tumors, such as the neuroblastoma. The sacrococcygeal teratoma occurs in three different forms: 1) an adult-mature form which is benign; 2) a mixed form, with mature and embryonal tissue, potentially malignant; and 3) an immature form represented by embryonal carcinoma, but also by neuroblastoma or adenocarcinoma.

Another classification is in relation; to the localization of the tumor: external, with glutei deformity (type 1); mainly external and in modest part internal (type 2); mainly internal (type 3); and only internal, inside the pelvis (type 4).

These lesions must be removed during the neonatal period: the dissection of the tumor capsula must be accomplished with caution, not to damage the fibers of the musculus levator ani, to avoid fecal incontinence. The coccyx must be completely removed, in case of benign tumors, in order to avoid relapses. In case of malignant tumors, the removal may be more complicated and the capsule must remain unbroken. The longer the operation is delayed, the more there are possibilities of a malignant transformation of the tumor, which can relapse or metastasize. In these cases we can apply chemotherapy, but its utility has not been proved.

10. Spinal tumors

Spinal tumors have various origins, but a common feature of their intrarachidian development is that they cause spinal or radicular compression or compression of the osteoligamentous structures of the vertebral canal. Spinal tumors can be distinguished in relation to their site of origin: extradural or rachidian tumors; intradural tumors: a) extramedullary and b) intramedullary.

Rachidian or extradural tumors

- *Osteogenetic tumors*
  Benign tumors: osteoma, osteoid osteoma, osteoblastoma, giant cell tumor.
  Malignant tumors: osteosarcoma, Ewing's sarcoma, myeloma.

- *Cartilaginous tumors*
  Benign tumors: chondroma, osteochondroma, chondroblastoma.
  Malignant tumors: chondrosarcoma.

- *Vascular tumors*
  Benign tumors: angioma, lymphagioma, angioreticuloma.
  Malignant tumors: angiosarcoma, hemangiopericytoma.

- *Connective tissue tumors*
  Benign tumors: fibroma, lipoma.
  Malignant tumors: fibrosarcoma, liposarcoma.

- Others tumors: metastases, chordoma.

Subdural extramedullary tumors

- Benign tumors: meningiomas, neurinomas, dermoid or epidermoid cysts, lipomas.
- Malignant tumors: metastases (rare).

Subdural intramedullary tumors

- Benign tumors: ependymomas, juvenile astrocytomas, angioreticulomas, dermoid or epidermoid cysts, choleostatomas, lipomas.
- Malignant tumors: anaplastic astrocytomas, glioblastomas, metastases (rare).

- **Frequency, gender, duration of the disease**
Frequency: meningiomas, neurinomas and intramedullary tumors represent more than 70% of neoplastic medullary compressions; 30% consists of extradural malignant tumors.
Gender: clear predominance of meningiomas in women.
Age: the average age is higher in meningiomas and extradural malignant tumors (51 years); the duration of the disease is variable.

Symptoms and signs

In about 70% of spinal tumors the first symptom consists in vertebral, radicular or cordonal pain followed by ordered by frequency motor disorders, sensory disorders, sphincteric and neurovegetative disorders, neurogenic intermittent claudication and subarachnoid hemorrhage.

Pain
Vertebral pain or rachiodynia is a dull and deep pain, limited to two or three contiguous vertebral segments. It is perceived in the vertebronuchal, infrascapular, dorsal or lumbar regions, with antalgic contracture of the paravertebral muscles. It is often associated with radicular or cordonal pain and it is more pronounced in extradural malignant tumors.
Radicular pain is a subcontinuous, gnawing ache, with sudden exacerbations, localized in the area of a sensitive spinal root. This pain is frequent and characteristic of extramedullary intradural tumors (60%-70% of

cases). It is rarer in extradural and intramedullary tumors, and it has a medullary origin, due to posterior horn irritation. It is perceived as burning, stinging, biting pain, without a strictly radicular distribution.

Cordonal pain is perceived as a painful disturbance, or as a diffuse burning or sharp sensation, spread in a segment of a limb or in part of the body; its characteristic is the progressively descending distribution. It is more frequent in intramedullary gliomas, especially cervical and dorsal. It can resemble an electric shock, similar to that caused by intraoperative stimulation of the posterior cordonal tracts.

Motor disturbance

This is the first and the most frequent symptom after pain and it is perceived as exhaustion and weakness of one or more limbs. It is due to the damage of one or more anterior roots, to the stress of the medullary anterior horns (ischemic damage) or to the involvement of the corticospinal tracts. In this last case the motor disturbance is spastic, while it is flaccid in the previous ones, although they can coexist.

Considering the disposition of fibers in the cruciate pyramidal tract (the fibers for the lower limbs are more external), the development of the motor deficit is ascending in extramedullary tumors and descending in intramedullary ones.

The evolution of meningiomas, neurinomas, and gliomas is slow and progressive, but it should be noted that apoplectiform onset, with transverse section syndrome or sudden deterioration, has been described in intramedullary, vertebral and malignant extradural tumors.

Paresthesias

They are persistent sensations of tingling, pricking, numbness and temperature extremes (hot or cold). They have variable distribution and spread along one or more limbs, thorax, and abdomen. They can have radicular or cornual, mono- or bilateral distribution. Similar to the motor deficit, paresthesias can have ascending progression in extramedullary tumors and descending progression in intramedullary tumors. They are unusual as an isolated initial symptom, but in meningiomas they are quite frequent (about 30% of cases).

Sensory deficits

They are reported as "dead skin" sensation, or loss of feeling in a finger or limb. The hypo-anesthesia can involve deep and/or superficial sensitivity, present a level or be suspended. It can have a cordonal distribution (due to ascending tract involvement) or metameric distribution (due to cornual or radicular involvement). The ascending evolution from more distal dermatomers in extramedullary tumors and descending evolution in intramedullary ones are quite relevant; the suspended hypo-anesthesia is almost pathognomonic of an intramedullary injury. As an isolated initial symptom they are unusual in all types of tumors.

Sphyncteric and sexual disorders

Impotentia erigendi and impotentia coeundi are unusual as initial symptoms. Sphincteric disorders are rare as well, with the exception of conus medullaris tumors.

Subarachnoid hemorrhage

It is quite unusual as a first symptom. The patient feels a sharp dorsal or dorsolumbar pain, without loss of consciousness. A meningeal syndrome is established with hemorrhagic cerebrospinal fluid.

Intermittent claudication

It is expression of medullary stress, and has been observed in some cases of vascular malformations and medullary hemangioblastomas. It is more frequent in lumbar canal stenosis and in vertebral column degenerative processes.

The necessity of an early diagnosis is incontrovertible, not only in the case of spinal tumors. 70% of spinal tumors begin with pain and 5%-20% begin with paresthetic-hypoesthetic disorders, i.e. with symptoms attributable to several other diseases, such as arthritis, neuritis, or visceral disorders. The second symptom is usually more clear and contributes to define an organic neurological syndrome (early syndrome, very little described in the literature). The frequency, association and type of disorders are different according to the location of the tumor.

Foramen magnum tumors

They are mainly represented by meningiomas, followed by neurinomas. The early syndrome is characterized by nuchal pain, often intense, radicular to C2 level (especially in neurinomas), paresthesias and/or paresis in one or both upper limbs with tetrahyperreflexia, more severe in the upper limbs. At the stage of status, hyposthenia in the hands is associated with atrophy of small muscles, spastic tetraparesis (more severe in the upper limbs), superficial and deep hypo-anesthesia irregularly distributed (sometimes with syringomyelic dissociation), hypoesthesia in the C2 territory, and sphincteric disorders. Sometimes deficits of the last cranial nerves and intracranial hypertension are present.

Cervical tumors

More than 50% of spinal tumors are meningiomas and neurinomas, followed by intramedullary tumors (about 30%) and extradural malignant tumors (6%-7%).

Neurinomas

They frequently arise from roots IV, V and VI while meningiomas mainly affect the higher cervical tract. The early syndrome is characterized by monoradicular unilateral, intense and continuous pain, occurring frequently at night, corresponding radicular sensitive deficit and initial motor disturbance. This syndrome is almost pathognomonic, although the soft or hard hernia can cause it. The differential diagnosis is easily done using plain films.

The symptoms and signs during the status stage are: muscular atrophies in radicular territory, Braun-Sequard's syndrome, hypo-anesthesia with level (more serious caudally), spastic paraparesis, and rare sphincteric disorders.

Meningiomas

During the precocious syndrome, they cause cordonal paresthesias in the lower limbs with a distal start, sometimes radicular pain and initial spastic mono-paraparesis. During the status stage, the clinical picture is characterized by paresis or mono-pluriradicular atrophy, Brown-Sequard's syndrome, serious spastic paraparesis, sensory disorders (more serious distally), and severe sphincteric disorders. This late clinical syndrome is almost identical to that of neurinoma. In fact, if the plain film shows widening of a conjugate foramen and, if cisternal hyperalbuminosis is found (frequent also in intramedullary hemangioblastomas), it is almost certainly a neurinoma.

Intramedullary tumors

During the early syndrome, when pain is present, it usually has cornual characteristics; radicular pain is rare. Cordonal pain in the upper limbs with slow descending development at the trunk and lower limbs has great diagnostic value. We can observe radicular paresis and mono- or bilateral atrophy in the upper limbs with fasciculations, radicular paresthesias, suspended hypoesthesia (pathognomonic), and hyperreflexia in the lower limbs.

During the status stage, we can observe serious paresis, spastic-flaccid atrophies in the upper limbs, often with fibrillations, spastic paraparesis, hypo-anesthesia (more serious proximally and with descending development), and rare sphincteric disorders.

Malignant extradural tumors

They are mainly represented by vertebral metastases (lung, prostate, breast), osteosarcamas, and Ewing's tumors. The *early syndrome* consists in vertebral pain and sharp pluriradicular pains, radicular paresthesias, initial spastic motor deficit in the lower limbs, flaccid-spastic motor deficit in the upper limbs, pluriradicular hypoesthesia in the upper limbs and/or cordonal in the lower limbs, and increased erythrocyte sedimentation rate. *During the status stage,* serious tetraparesis (spastic-flaccid in the upper limbs) occurs, associated with level hypoanesthesia (more serious distally) and sphincteric disorders.

Dorsal tumors

The dorsal and the lumbosacral spinal cord are the medullary tracts most frequently affected by spinal tumors. In fact, 70%-85% of meningiomas develop at dorsal level, with clear predominance in women (80%); the neurinomas represent 40%-51%, the malignant extradural tumors 60% (above all metastases). In children sarcomas and sympatoblastomas are frequent. Gliomas have an incidence between 40% and 58%.

Neurinomas

The early syndrome is characterized by monoradicular, mono- or bilateral pain, often reproducing a visceral pain, and by radicular hypoesthesia, and spastic paraparesis associated or not with cordonal sensitive deficit. The late stage is characterized by a Brown-Séquard's syndrome, spastic paraparesis, bilateral hypo-anesthesia with level (more serious distally) and sphincteric disorders. This slow syndrome is almost analogous to meningiomas and malignant extradural tumors.

Meningiomas

The early syndrome is characterized by vertebral and radicular pain, cordonal paresthesias with distal onset in the lower limb, mono- or bilateral distal hypoesthesias, and slight monoparaparesis. During the status phase, there are, as in neurinomas, Brown-Séquard's syndrome, bilateral hypo-anesthesia with level (more serious distally), serious spastic paraparesis, and sphincteric disorders.

Malignant extradural tumors

The *early syndrome* consists in strong pain, mainly vertebral, but also radicular or pluriradicular (mono- or bilateral, "belt like"), which often can resemble visceral pains. There is an increase in the erythrocyte sedimentation rate. Afterwards, we can observe abrupt ingravescent paraparesis, bilateral hypo-anesthesia with level (more serious distally) and sphincteric disorders.

Intramedullary tumors

The *early syndrome* consists in descending pain in the thorax and/or abdomen, cordonal and vertebral pain, rarely radicular or cornual pain, sometimes fasciculations of dorsal muscle, suspended hypo-anesthesia, and spastic mono-paraparesis. *During the status phase*, spastic mono-paraparesis, level hypo-anesthesia, and sphincteric disorders are present.

Cono-filum tumors

Neurinomas

In *the early syndrome,* a sciatic radicular pain with negative Lasegue's sign is common. Pain is associated with motor disorder of spastic-flaccid type in one or both lower limbs with fasciculations, and radicular or cordonal hypoesthesia with regular distribution.

The initial pain can have the character of an abdomino-inguinal neuralgia or cruralgia, quite frequent in gliomas.

The status phase is characterized by a flaccid and/or spastic motor deficit in the lower limbs, cordonal and/or radicular sensory deficit, mainly "saddle" sensory deficiency, and sphincteric disorders.

Meningiomas

Lumbar meningiomas are rare. *During the early syndrome,* mono- or bilateral radicular pain occurs; it can rarely spread as sciatalgia, even bilaterally. We can observe radicular or cordonal paresthesias, hypotonia and hypodynamia in the lower limbs, often with fasciculations, and mild sensitive, pluriradicular or metameric deficits. When the medullary conus is involved, sexual and sphincteric disorders can be present. *During the status phase,* spastic-flaccid paraparesis occurs, with hypo-anesthesia in the lower limbs, more serious at the saddle (it can also appear in the early stage), and sphincteric disorders.

Malignant extradural tumors

The early syndrome is characterized by intense vertebral and pluriradicular pains, flaccid and/or spastic paresis, pluriradicular or level sensory deficit and increased erythrocyte sedimentation rate.

In the status phase, serious flaccid paraparesis, level hypo-anesthesia, and sphincteric disorders can be observed.

Intramedullary tumors

The early syndrome is often characterized by a pseudosciatalgia in form of nocturnal, indeterminate pain, of cornual origin, with negative Lasegue's sign.

Often it is intermittent and considered typical of a disk herniation, but it is often observed in oncogenic sciatalgias as well; fasciculations are found in the lower limbs, with spastic-flaccid motor deficit and irregular distribution.

In the status phase, flaccid-spastic paraparesis occurs with atrophies in the lower limbs, "patch" hypo-anesthesia, sometimes with syringomyelic dissociation and sphincteric disorders.

Radiological diagnosis

In intramedullary tumors, the plain films can show erosion of the peduncle and increase of the interpeduncalar distance at multiple levels. In neurinomas, the plain film can show erosion of the peduncles, which rarely overcome the extension of a vertebra, erosion of the posterior surface of the vertebral body, and enlargment of a conjugate foramen. These features allow the formulation of a diagnosis (Fig. 10.1).

In the meningioma, the bony alterations are less frequent and are limited at the peduncle of only one vertebra. In hemangioblastoma, the radiographic examination can show peduncular erosion and widening of the canal. In vertebral angioma, the radiographic examination shows a typical "courduroy cloth" aspect. In metastatic tumors, the examination shows osteolytic or osteoblastic alterations.

At present, the radiological diagnosis is based on computerized imaging (CT and NMR). The greater utility of CT or NMR depends on the characteristics of the tumor. In general, NMR, considering its excellent method of image formation and the possibility of obtaining multiplanar and panoramic images of the whole neuraxis, is the best choice. CT is mainly useful in tumors departing from the bone or in cases in which the osseous reworking is expression of the tumoral evolution.

The extramedullary intradural tumors are mainly meningiomas and neurinomas. In these tumors, spinal CT is important (but always complementary to NMR) only in cases of neurinomas of notable dimensions, in which the bony erosion is an important element for diagnosis (Fig. 10.1) and surgical planning. In the other cases, the best method is NMR, which, in neurinomas, shows an iso-hypointense lesion on T1-weighted images with marked enhancement with gadolinium and a hyperintense lesion on T2-weighted images (Fig. 10.6). In meningiomas, the NMR findings are similar to the previous ones (the diagnosis of the nature of the lesion often is not easy), even if the enhancement with gadolinium is less marked and sometimes the lesion in T2 appears isointense rather than hyperintense (Figs. 10.3; 10.4).

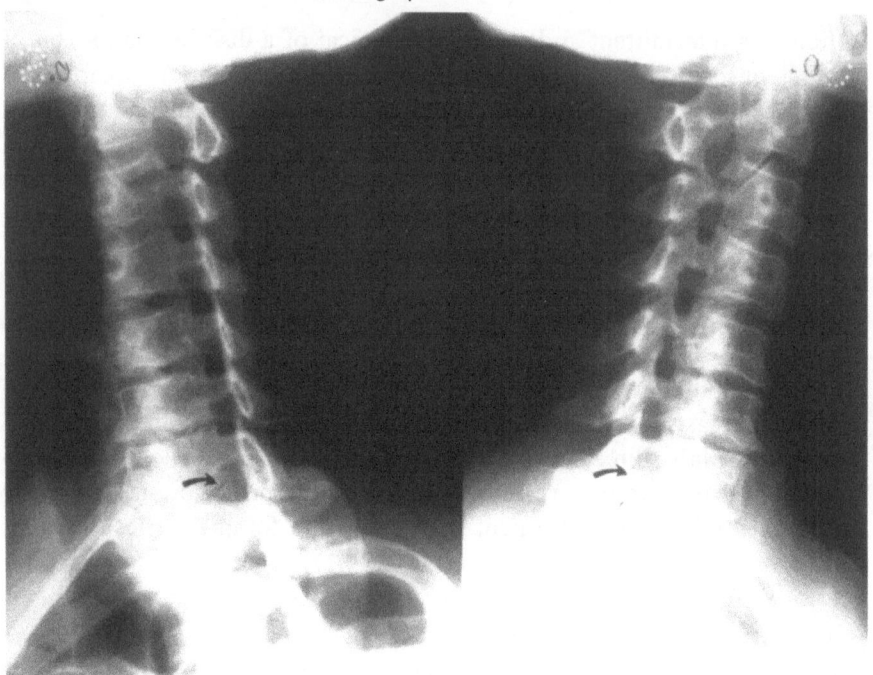

a

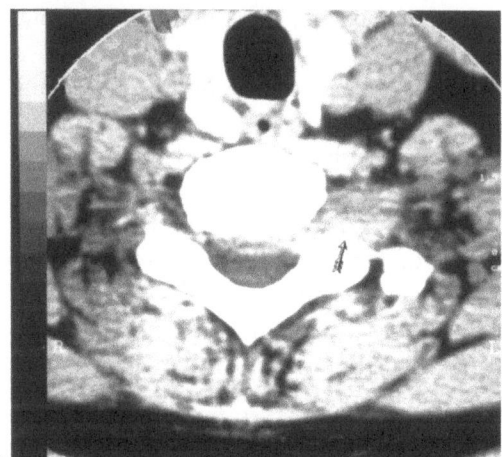

b

Fig. 10.1a,b. Left C7-D1 neurinoma. Cervical X-ray, oblique view (a): widening of the right conjugate foramen. Cervical CT (b): pathological tissue in the left intra-extra-foraminal region

The rare spinal dermoid cyst (extramedullary intradural) is hypodense on CT but on NMR it has a variable aspect, and is frequently iso-hyperintense on all sequences.

In extradural tumors, which are mostly bone tumors with secondary involvement of the epidural space and eventual myelo-radicular compres-

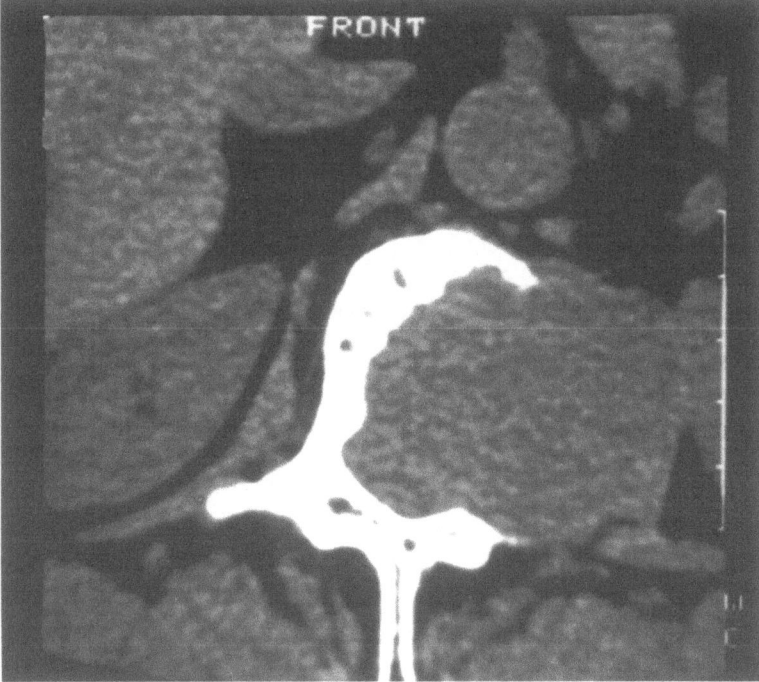

Fig. 10.2. Vertebral metastasis. Baseline CT scan focused at D11 level. Presence of pathological tissue which causes a vast osteolysis of the D11 vertebral body half, peduncle and transverse apophysis. The lesion extends into the vertebral canal and presses the spinal cord

sion, CT has an important diagnostic value. In relation to the osseous reworking caused by the tumor, CT images change according to the presence of osteoblastic, osteolytic or mixed lesions (as observed in some mammary or prostatic metastases) (Fig. 10.2). In the first case, the lesions appear hyperdense, while the ostelytic lesions appear hypodense. The mixed lesions, more frequently found, will have a mixed hyper- and hypodense aspect. With NMR, osteoblastic lesions appear hypointense on T1-weighted images, while osteolytic lesions appear mainly iso-hypointense on T1 and hyperintense on T2. In the lipoma, an expansive lesion mainly extradural and often associated with congenital malformations of spinal dysraphism, NMR, on the contrary of osseous tumors, has an essential role for the diagnosis. It shows a lesion iso-hypointense on T1 and hyperintense on T2 (Fig. 10.7).

The intramedullary tumors are essentially of glial nature, mainly astrocytomas and ependymomas. In these types of tumor, CT is useless for the

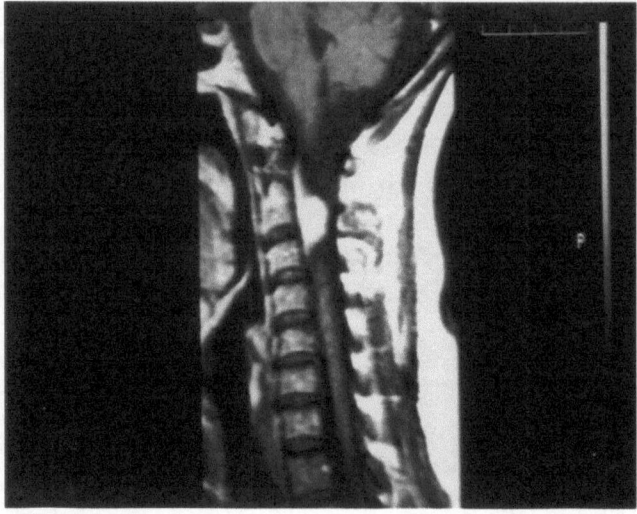

Fig. 10.3. Cervical meningioma. NMR, T1-weighted image, after contrast medium administration, sagittal view. Presence of tissue characterized by a marked and homogeneous contrast enhancement at the level of the spinal canal anterior aspect with extension from C1 to C3. A meningeal contrast enhancement and spinal cord compression are present

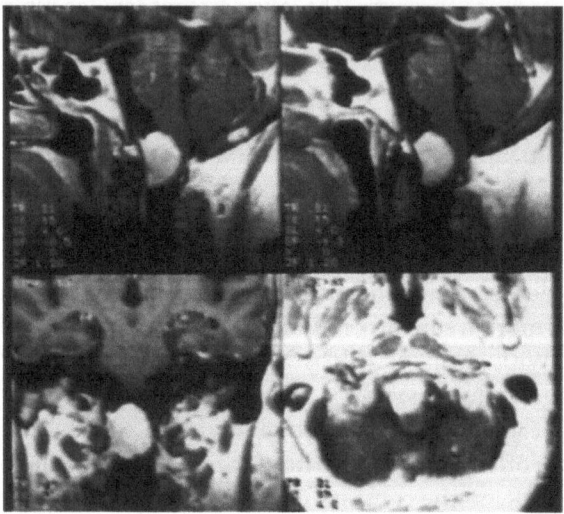

Fig. 10.4. Meningioma of the craniospinal junction. Cerebral NMR, T1-weighted images, axial, coronal and sagittal views after contrast medium administration. Neoformation with marked and homogeneous contrast enhancement, with dural anterior point of origin and compression on the spinal cord and bulb

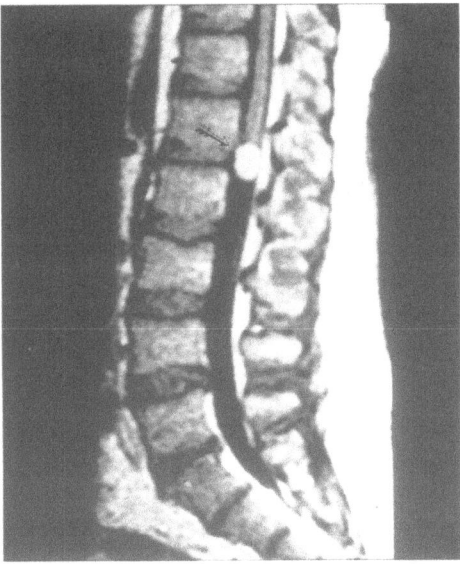

Fig. 10.5. Lumbar neurinoma. NMR, T1-weighted image, after contrast medium administration. Presence of pathological tissue into the vertebral canal, at the level of the posterior aspect of the L1-L2 disk, with marked and homogeneous contrast enhancement

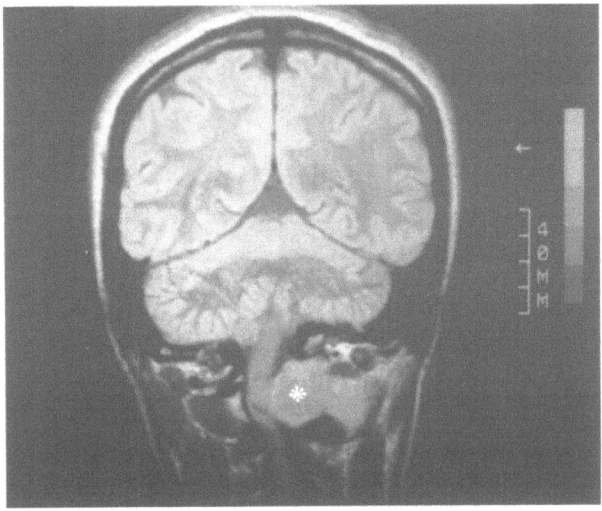

Fig. 10.6. Left C1-C2 neurinoma. NMR, T1-weighted image, coronal view. Large intra-extradural mass with vast osteolysis and spinal cord compression

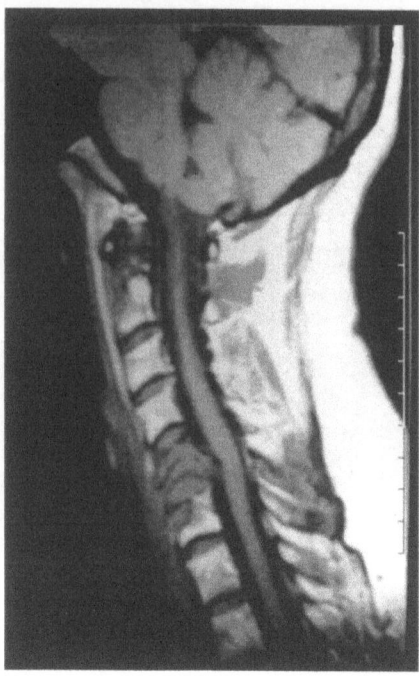

Fig. 10.7. Vertebral metastasis. NMR, T1-weighted image, sagittal view. Presence of a C5-C6 vertebral body morpho-structural and signal alterations and spinal cord ventral surface compression

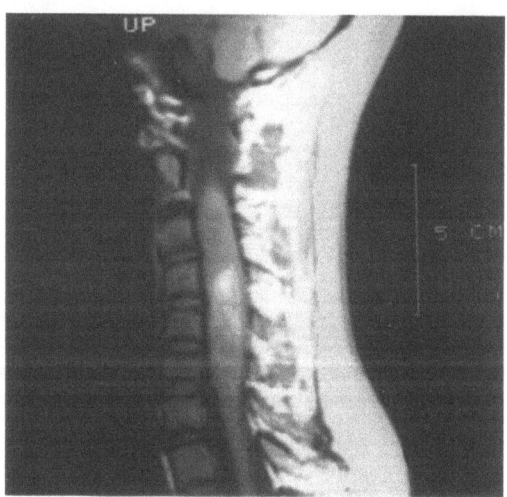

Fig. 10.8. Cervical intra-medullary astrocytoma. NMR, T1-weighted image, sagittal view

diagnosis. NMR shows, in the majority of cases, iso-hypointense lesions on T1 and hyperintense lesions on T2, with enhancement after gadolinum (Fig. 10.8).

The differential diagnosis of these tumors is still a discussed subject. Even though various diagnostic-differential criteria between astrocytoma and intramedullary ependymoma have been elaborated, such as the enhancement modalities (more intense, homogenous and limited in ependymomas) or the appearance of peritumoral hypointensity (more frequent in ependymomas), it is still not possible to formulate a certain radiological preoperative diagnosis.

This differential diagnosis is exclusively histological and, being essential to decide the grade of tumor removal (presence of cleavage plane in the ependymoma, often absent in the astrocytoma, allowing a more frequent total removal), the extemporaneous biopsy of the tumor during surgery is always indicated.

In the hemangioblastoma, NMR shows a dyshomogeneous iso-hypointense mass on T1-weighted images and a hyperintense mass on T2, with clear enhancement after endovenous gadolinium injection. In 50% of the cases, serpiginous flow-void areas are found.

Surgical therapy and prognosis

Therapy for spinal tumors is surgical and consists in the removal of the pathological tissue that compresses the nervous structures (nerve roots and spinal cord) and alters their functions. The prognosis depends on tumoral histology, early diagnosis, and the location and extent of the tumor.

Intradural extramedullary tumors

The intradural extramedullary tumors (neurinomas, meningiomas) are always removable, with possible functional recovery and definitive healing (Figs. 10.9; 10.10).

Intramedullary tumors

The prognosis of intramedullary tumors has clearly improved since the introduction, in the surgical procedures, of the surgical microscope, bipo-

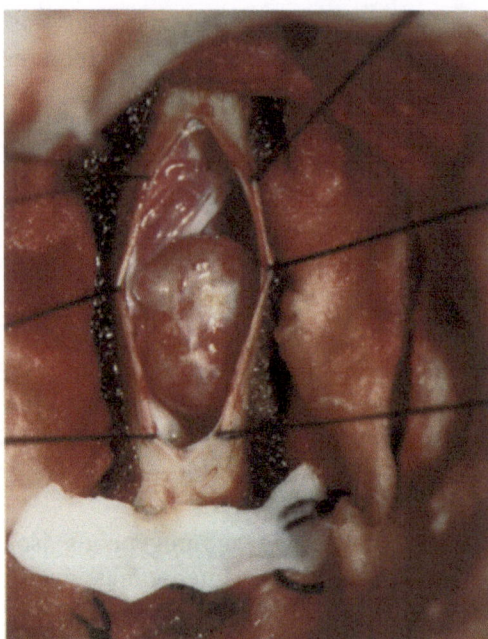

Fig. 10.9. Surgical aspect of an intradural extramedullary meningioma

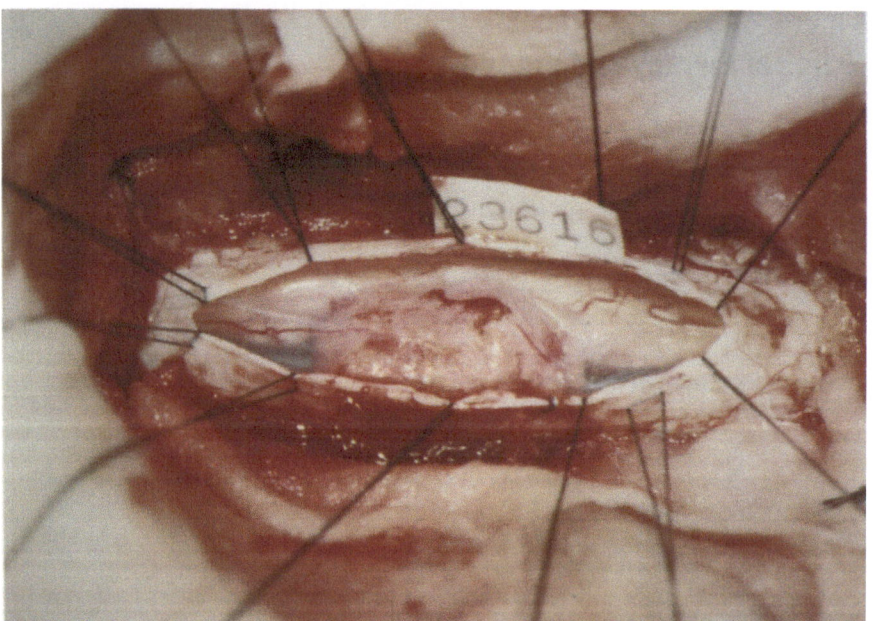

Fig. 10.10. Surgical aspect of an intradural extramedullary neurinoma

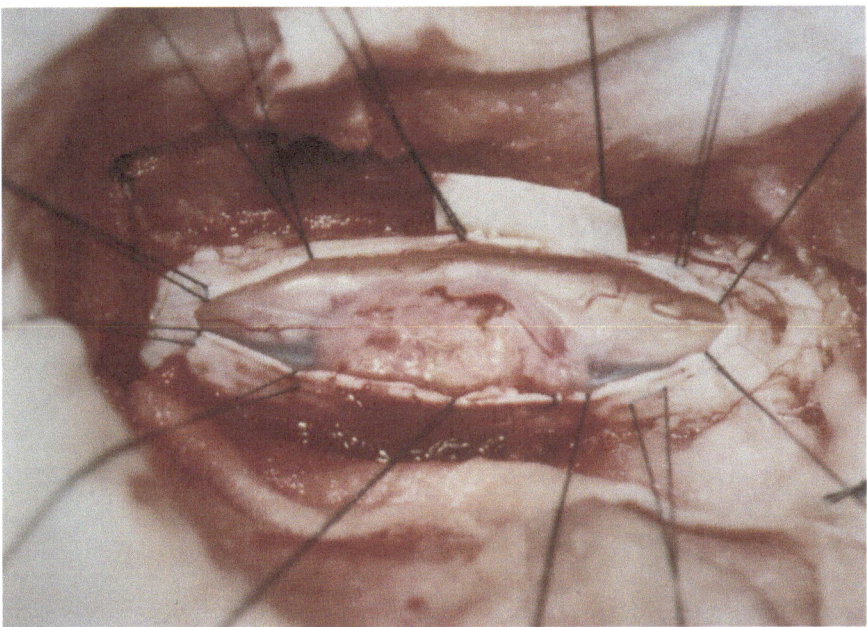

Fig. 10.11. Surgical aspect of an intramedullary ependymoma

lar coagulation, cavitron, and LASER. In intramedullary noninfiltrating tumors (ependymomas, hemangioblastomas, juvenile astrocytomas), radical removal is possible with definitive healing. In intramedullary infiltrating tumors (astrocytomas, glioblastomas, lipomas), removal can only be partial with consequent relapse (Fig. 10.11).

Extradural tumors

The majority of extradural tumors consists in malignant neoplasias, generally metastases from carcinomas. The therapeutic approach must be multidisciplinary: surgical, radiotherapeutic and chemotherapeutic. The aim of the surgical procedure is to decompress the spinal cord and nerve roots and to stabilize the vertebral column with metallic devices and acrylic material.

The prognosis depends on the histology: in malignant lesions the regression of the symptomatology is transient, but it is definitive in benign lesions.

11. Spinal cord vascular malformations

Vascular malformation myelopathies

These dysembryogenetic malformations, also called medullary angiomas, are dilations or anomalies of the arterial, venous or capillary vascular compartment. We distinguish: the *raceme-venous angioma* (exclusively of venous nature), formed by bluish pial vein conglomerates, sinuous, not pulsating, containing venous blood, and sometimes an ample more or less tortuous vein; and the *arteriovenous angioma*, formed by arteries and veins communicating between them through a tangle of abnormal vessels, without capillary interposition. This angioma appears as a turgid group of pulsating arteria vessels, containing high pressure arterial blood and by ample, tortuous, venous vessels, pulsating as well; the *arterial angioma*, purely arterial, is very rare in the spinal cord; the *cavernous angiomas or cavernomas* are tumor-like malformations of small dimensions, without intervascular tissue, often they are surrounded by coagulated venous blood; the *telangectasias* are dilations of capillary vessels separated by normal tissue. They can have cavernomatous aspect due to progressive dilation of the vasal walls and secondary disappearance of intervascular tissue.

The most affected medullar segments are, according to frequency, the medio-inferior dorsal, lumbar, and cervical segments. The angiomas are more frequent in men during the third through fifth decades of life, and are associated with cutaneous angiomas, often corresponding to the affected neuromere or neuromeres of other areas (brain, pons), or with other malformations (syringomyelia, spina bifida).

Clinically, we may observe: 1) deficitary or radicular syndrome, due to compressive action on the posterior spinal roots; the pain is sudden, lancinating, similar to a cervicobrachial neuralgia, intercostal neuralgias (sometimes simulating a visceropathy), cruralgias and sciatalgias. The pain can increase or appear during decubitus; often sensory or motor deficits are associated, with radicular distribution. 2) Acute transverse myelopathy syndrome is due to an intramedullar hemorrhage or to spinal necrosis caused by rupture or thrombosis of an anomalous vessel; we can observe blood diffusion in the subarachnoid spaces, with corresponding subarachnoid hemorrhage syndrome. 3) Syndrome of progressive medullary compression or radiculo-medullary syndrome, less characteristic than the previous ones. The clinical picture of the different medullary syndromes is in relation to their localization; a cervicodorsolumbar clinical syndrome occurs when the malformation involves the entire spinal cord. At each level, the sensorimotor deficits can have multiform and bizarre features, appearing not to be due to a single focus. The clinical course is chronic, subcontinuous, with remissions and excerbations of the symptomatology. Even in

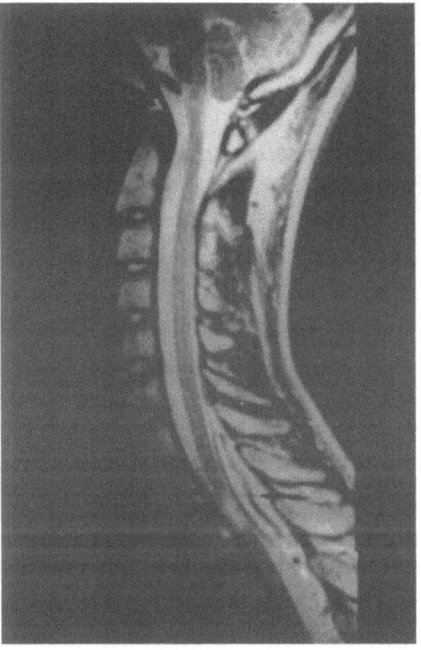 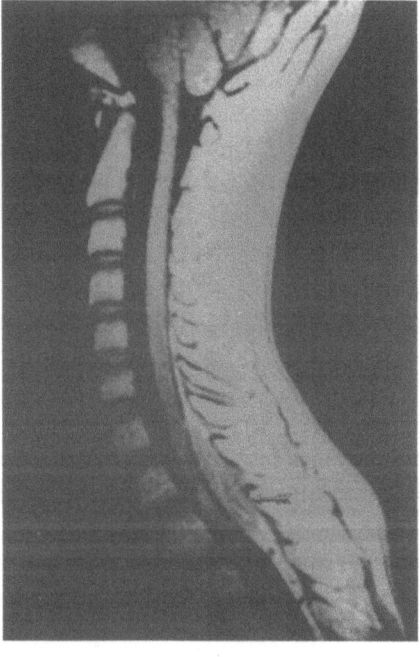

a b

Fig. 11.1a,b. Spinal arteriovenous malformations. NMR, T1-weighted (**a**) and T2-weighted (**b**) images, sagittal views. Epidural hematic collection extends from C7 to D3, in its context a structure of tubular morphology and absence of signal is present. This is expression of vascular malformation. The epidural hematoma causes a compression on the spinal cord in which a hyperintense zone of distress is present on the T2-weighted image

cases of transverse syndrome, there can be a more or less complete remission of the symptoms. The rachicentesis, in the majority of cases, is normal; in 15%-20% of cases it can point out a manometric block with albuminocytologic dissociation and hemorrhagic cerebrospinal fluid. NMR shows the malformation as serpiginous vessels with absence of signal on T1- and T2-weighted images, with the veins more ample and recognizable

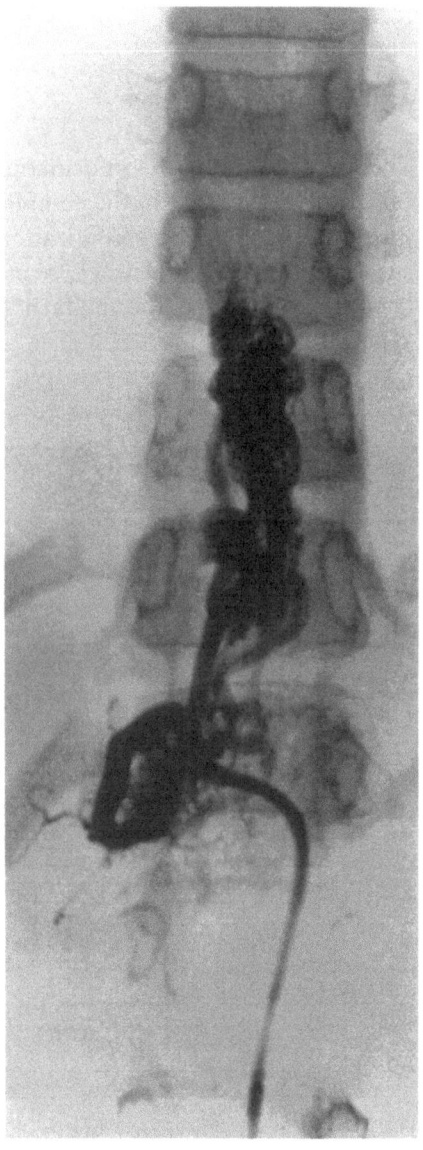

Fig. 11.2. Dorsolumbar spinal angiography. Selective angiography of the right dilatated intercostal artery. A spinal angioma at D9-D10 level is fed by the intercostal artery

than the arteries. It also shows the anterior or posterior location of the malformation, its size, and the possible presence of an intramedullar hemorrhagic focus. This focus is hyperintense in subacute and chronic stages, while it is isointense or slightly hypointense, in the acute stage (Fig. 11.1). Spinal angiography is essential for proper treatment and should be done after NMR. Angiography shows the angioma in its different aspects: dilated afferent arteries, tangled vessels and dilated drain veins (Fig. 11.2).

Computed myelotomography shows vascular tortuosity.

Therapy

Therapy is based on the information provided by angiography. The surgical treatment consists in the complete removal of the malformation, sometimes preceded by the embolization of arterial afferences to facilitate the surgical intervention (Fig. 11.3). In some cases, an accurate embolization completely obstructs the malformation, rendering the surgical operation superfluous.

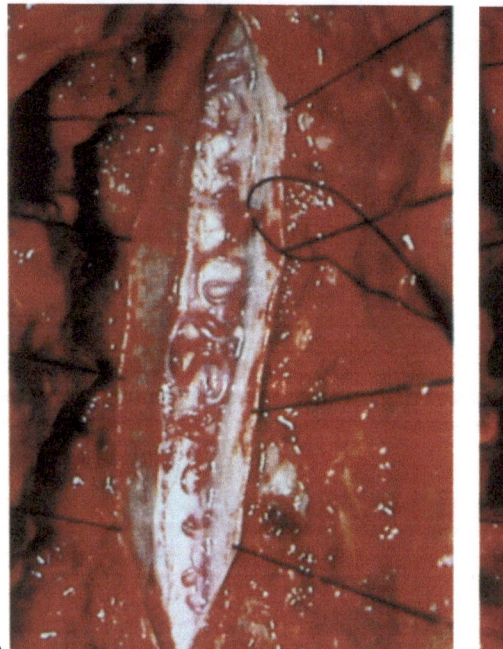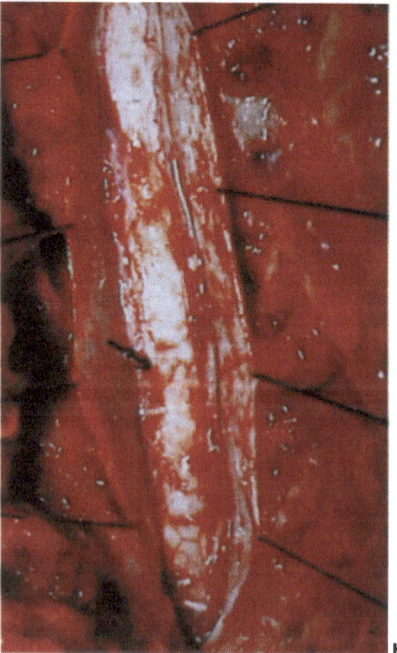

a   b

Fig. 11.3a,b. Pre-operative (**a**) and postoperative (**b**) aspects of a spinal angioma

12. Pathology of disk degeneration

The intervertebral disk is a proper intersomatic joint between two vertebrae, allowing pluridirectional movements. The disk, composed of the pulposus and gelatinous nucleus with collagen fibers and contained inside a fibrous ring, changes its morphology during movements of the column. The intervertebral disks are maintained in place by the two anterior and posterior longitudinal ligaments, which are also the longitudinal union means of the vertebral bodies.

Disk pathology is represented by disk herniation and spondylosis. Disk herniation is due to softening of the fibrous ring (contained hernia, Fig. 12.1) or its breakage (excluded hernia, Fig. 12.2, migrated hernia, Fig. 12.3), with the displacement of the nucleus polposus in posterior, postero-lateral or lateral direction (Figs. 12.4-12.7).

Spondylosis is a secondary disease, consequence of a plurimetameric chronic disk pathology. The disks are flattened and, because of the contiguous vertebral body friction, a reactive osteogenesis is stimulated along the vertebral body margin, with osteophyte formation. These osteophytes tighten the conjugation canals (irritative and deficitary radicular disorders) and posterior ones, projecting in the vertebral canal, reduce its diameter (myelopathies) (Figs. 12.8; 12.9).

Cervical disk herniation

It is less frequent than lumbar disk herniation. It can occur at any age and it is often a consequence of sudden stress on the neck, directly or passively inflicted, as in a car crash (acute hernia, whiplash injury).

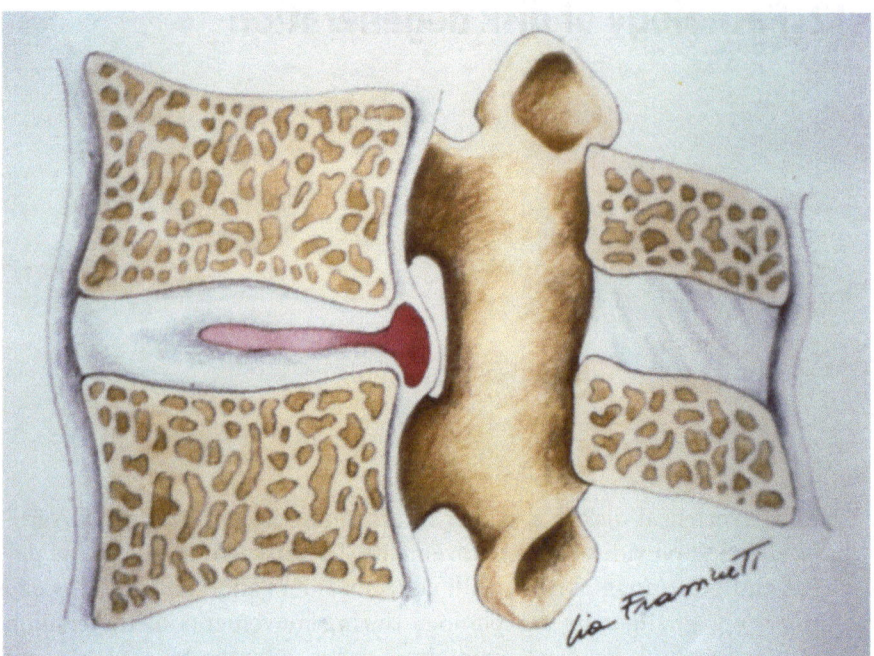

Fig. 12.1. Contained hernia

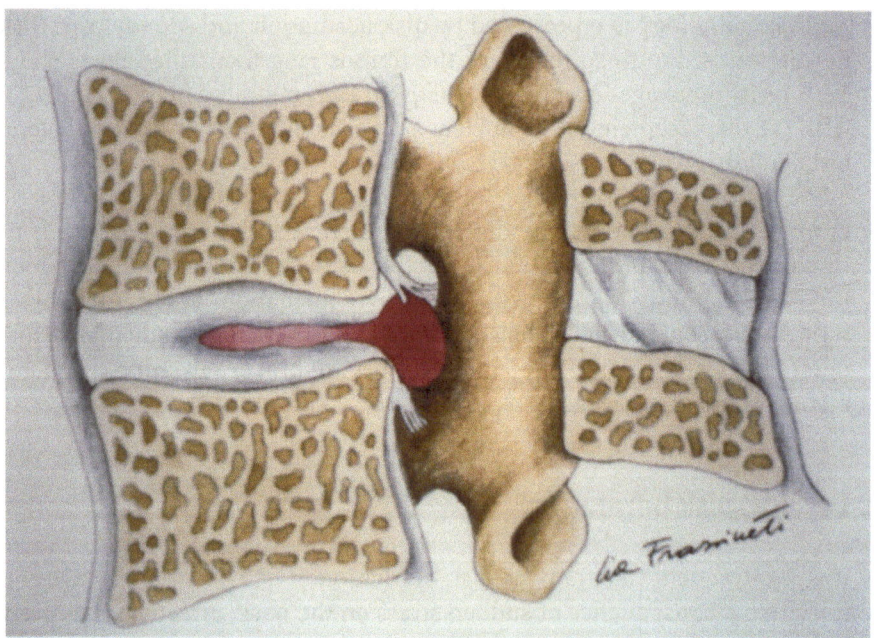

Fig. 12.2. Excluded hernia

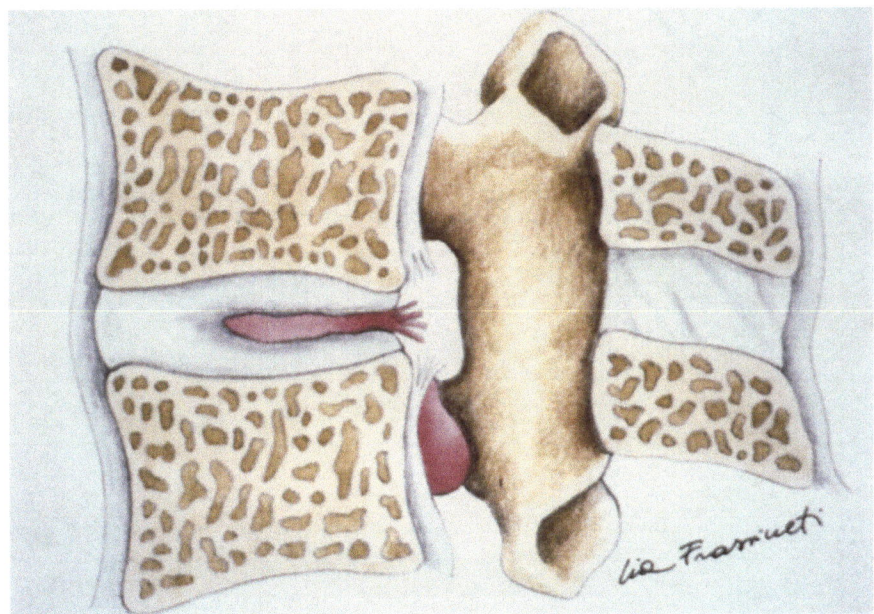

Fig. 12.3. Migrated hernia

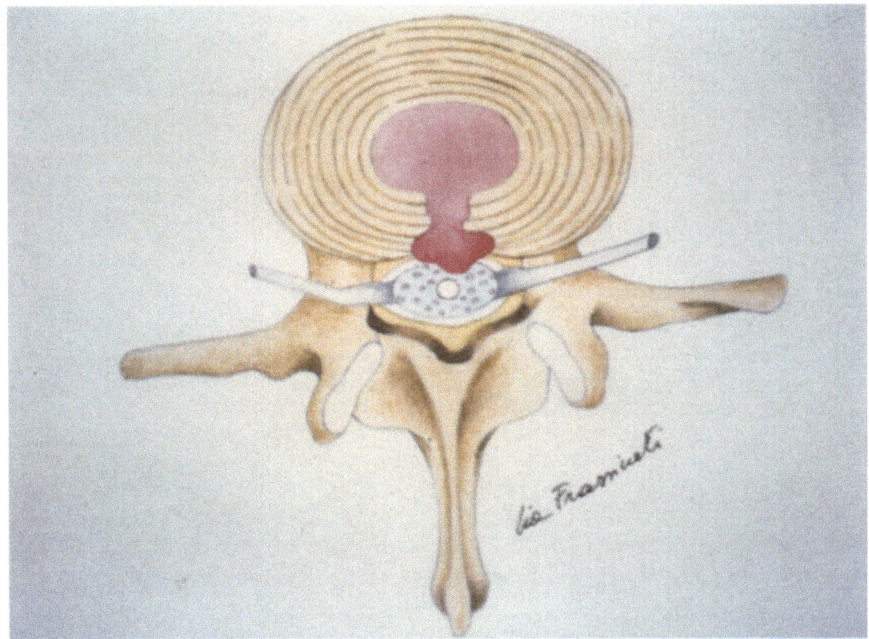

Fig. 12.4. Median lumbar disk herniation

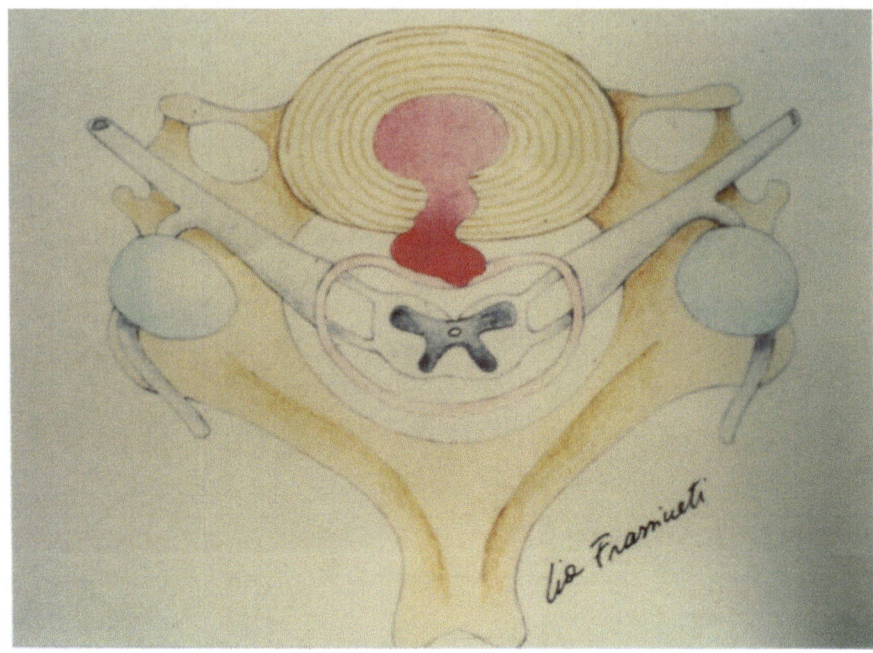

Fig. 12.5. Median cervical disk herniation with medullar compression

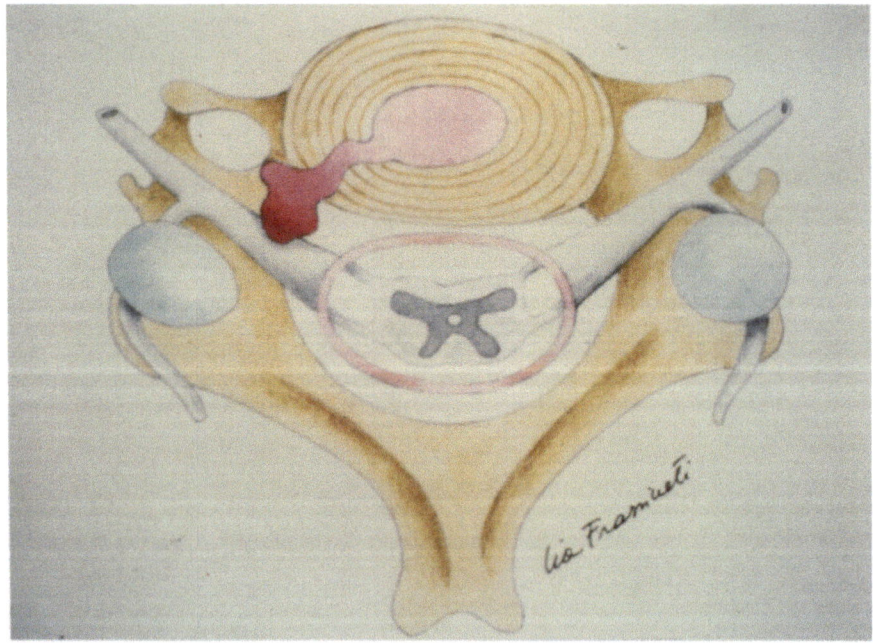

Fig. 12.6. Cervical lateral disk herniation with radicular compression

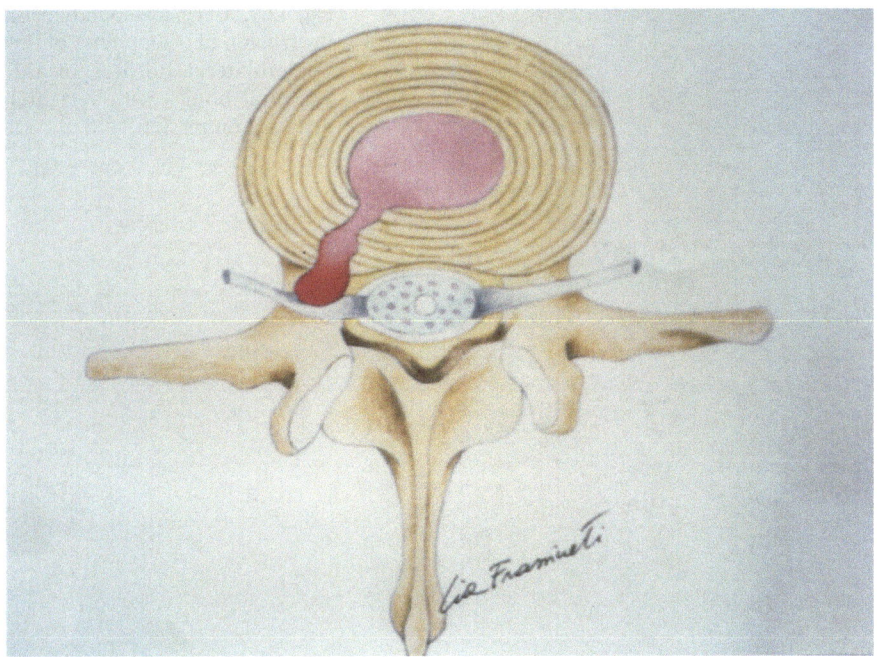

Fig. 12.7. Lateral lumbar disk herniation with intraforaminal radicular compression

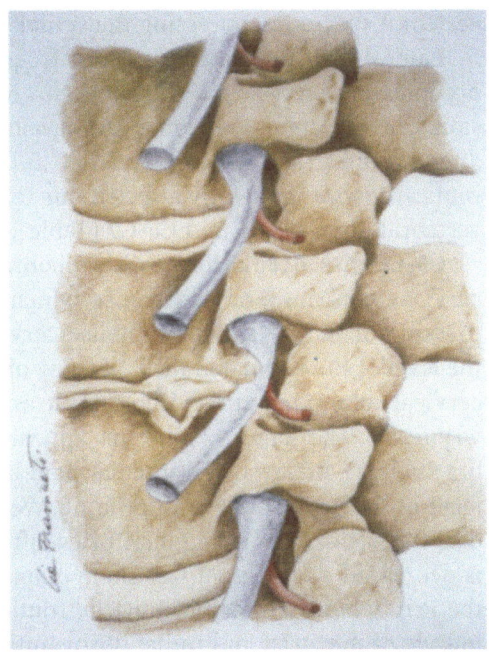

Fig. 12.8. Cervical spondylosis: bulging of posterolateral osteophytes of the vertebral bodies with decreased area of intervertebral foramina and nerve root compression

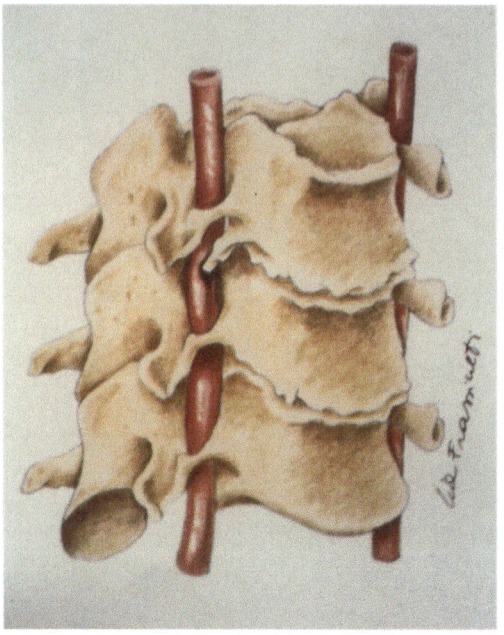

Fig. 12.9. Cervical spondylosis: protrusion of osteophytes of the posterolateral borders of the vertebral bodies with vertebral artery compression

Median disk herniation can be central and may partially occupy the vertebral specus, compressing the spinal cord.

Lateral disk herniation is more frequent than the previous one, and occupies the recessi and conjugate foramina, causing radicular compression. The radicular syndrome can develop slowly or suddenly, sometimes after a trauma (soft hernia). The C6 (C5-C6 hernia) and C7 (C6-C7 hernia) roots are more frequently affected due to the greater mobility of the intervertebral disks C5-C6 and C6-C7 (Table 12.1).

C5-C6 disk herniation (C6 cervicobrachialgia) occurs with a sudden cervical pain, more or less intense, which gradually decreases in time. The pressing of the neck causes intense cervical pain, sometimes stronger at the level of the herniated disk. We may observe symmetric or asymmetric cervical column rigidity with scoliotic antalgic attitude (diskal herniation wryneck). The same symptoms appear in C6-C7 hernia (C7 cervicobrachialgia). Afterwards, radicular pain irradiates to the anterolateral surfaces of the arm, forearm and thumb. We may also observe sensory disorders in the corresponding territories, often paresthesias, the biceps reflex is decreased or absent, a faradic hypoexcitability of the biceps muscle of the arm, anterior brachial muscle, round pronator muscle, radial flexor muscle of the wrist and radial flexor muscles of the thumb.

Tab. 12.1.

Herniation level	Root involved	Pain and paresthesia radiation	Motor deficits	Reflex deficits
C5-C6	C6	Deltoid, lateral arm, forearm, thumb	Biceps	Biceps
C6-C7	C7	Posterior arm, forearm, hand dorsum, middle finger	Triceps, extensor digitorum	Triceps
C7-T1	C8	Medial arm, forearm, fourth and little finger	Hand intrinsic muscles	Sthiloradial
L3-L4	L4	Lateral gluteus, thigh, anterior leg	Quadriceps	Knee
L4-L5	L5	Posterior gluteus, thigh, lateral leg, foot dorsum, hallux	Extensor hallucis, extensor digitorum	None
L5-S1	S1	Posterior gluteus, thigh, leg, foot sole, fifth finger	Triceps surae, flexor hallucis	Ankle, medioplantar

C6-C7 disk herniation (C7 cervicobrachialgia) causes pain irradiating along the forearm cubital margin and last two fingers, mainly the little finger. Interosseal muscles are involved and, in part, those of the thenar eminence.

C4-C5 disk herniation (C5 cervicobrachialgia) causes pain in the scapulohomeral region. Deltoid muscle hypotrophy is present.

C3-C4 disk herniation (C4 cervicobrachialgia) causes pain limited to the scapular region. The cervical spine plain film may be normal, but in about 60% of cases it shows a narrowing of the intervertebral space, corresponding to the herniated disk. This narrowing is usually regular and associated with anterior and posterior marginal exostosis (modest for the most part, but sometimes more evident). Another recurrent radiographic sign is the decrease or disappearance of the physiological lordosis. CT shows a hypodense median or lateral disk image, protruding in the spinal canal or foramen. NMR shows an intrarachidian injury, anterior to the spinal cord, iso-hypointense on T1-weighted images and more hypointense on T2-weighted images (Figs. 12.10; 12.11a,b).

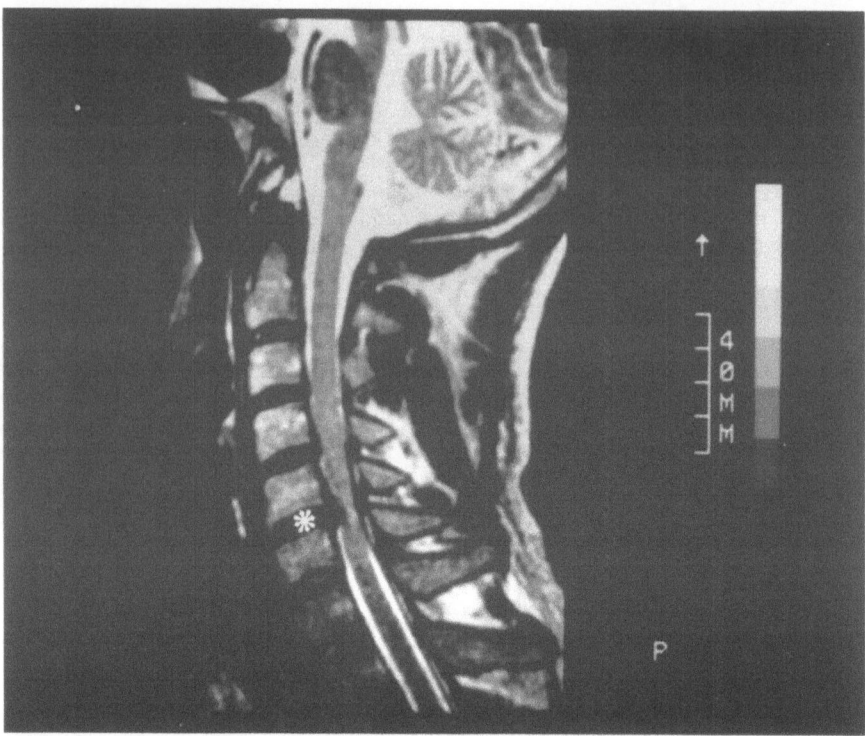

Fig. 12.10. Cervical disk herniation. NMR, T2-weighted image, sagittal view. Tissue of diskal intensity, localized at C5-C6 level compressing the ventral surface of the spinal cord

Therapy

Some patients (i.e. those with small hernias, bearable pain) initially can improve by using a neck immobilization collar, analgesics and muscle relaxants. In other cases presenting neurological deficits (middle-large hernias, intense pain), surgical therapy is necessary, using an anterior or posterior approach with disk removal.

Dorsal disk herniation

They are very rare. Considering that the spatial relationship between disks and roots is tight (the roots enter the conjugate foramina within a few millimeters of the emergence), radicular compression syndromes are unusual. Clinically they appear with intercostal, abdominal, and inguinal neuralgias, often attribuited to visceropathies. The medullary compression syndrome

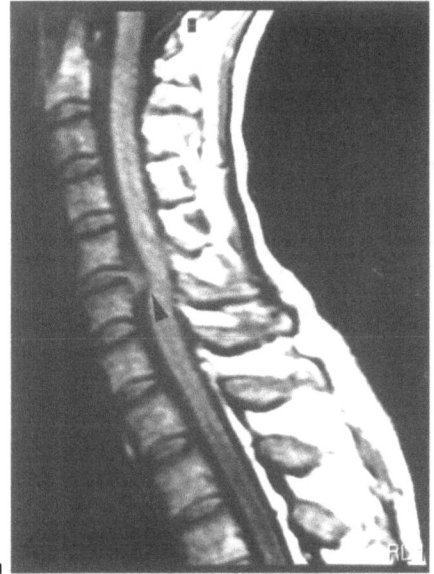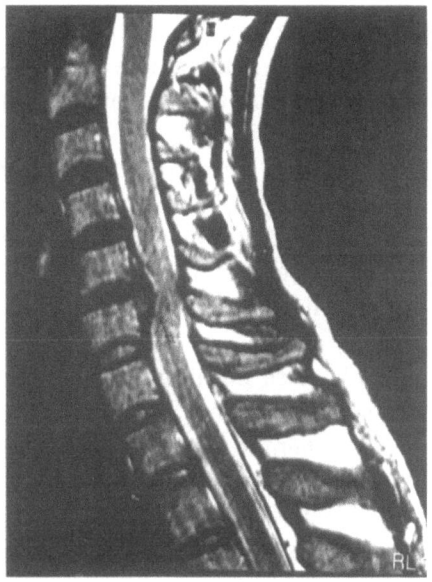

a   b

Fig. 12.11a,b. Cervical disk herniation. NMR, sagittal view, T1-weighted image (a) and T2-weighted image (b). Presence of an extensive tissue, with signal similar to that of a disk, at C5-C6 level with posterior spinal cord compression and displacement

has a slow development and it is not peculiar: it may begin with spastic paraparesis, ascending hypo-anesthesia and sphincterial disorders. The dorsal spine X-rays show the narrowing of a diskal space and the nucleus pulposus calcifications at the level of the medullary compression.

The diagnosis is possible with NMR, which shows an iso-hypointense hernia on T1-weighted images and a hypointense lesion on T2-weighted images. It can also show a hyperintense area on T2-weight images due to medullary parenchymal stress.

The therapy is surgical, with an anterolateral or posterolateral approach, which allows easy disk removal and reduces the iatrogenic neurological risks.

Lumbar disk herniation

Lumbar disk herniation, in 96%-98% of cases, compresses and stretches one or more roots by a direct mechanism. This happens more often along the extradural tract (the "radicular nerve"), but sometimes in the intradural tract as well, causing both vertebral (symmetric or asymmetric lumbar rigidity with antalgic attitudes in scoliosis, in kiphosis, in hyperlordosis, and vertebral pain), and radicular symptoms which, according to the disk involved, can occur with various clinical syndromes (Fig. 12.12).

L3-L4 disk herniation. Pain irradiates to the territory of the femoral nerve, and the thigh is in semiflexion with a positive Wasserman's sign. We can observe hypoesthesia or anesthesia of the third medium or inferior of the thigh, patellar hypo-areflexia, rarely normoreflexia, thigh hypotrophy and faradic hypoexcitability of the corresponding myomeres.

L4-L5 disk herniation. It is the most frequent herniation and it can cause two syndromes:
1) *L5 monoradicular sciatalgia* is the most common form, mainly due to a lateral herniation. Pain is irradiated along the posterior surface of the thigh until the poples, and along the antero-external surface of the leg until the back of the foot. We can observe: normoreflexia and light or absent hypotrophy of the leg, often a decrease in strength of the dorsal

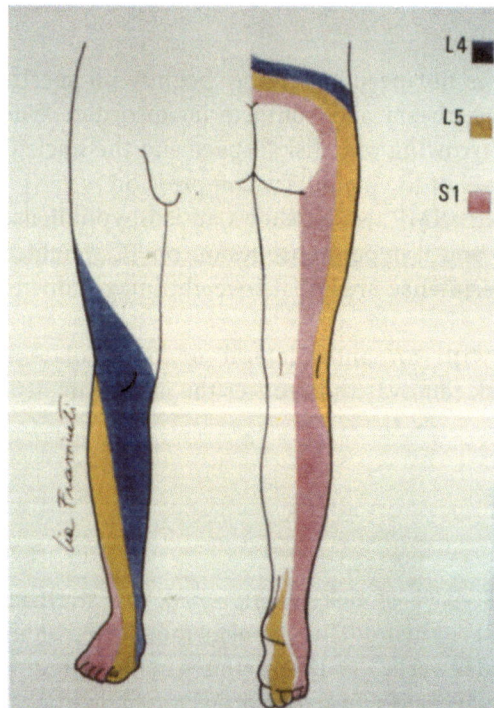

Fig. 12.12. Pain radiation area along the dematomere corresponding to the involved root

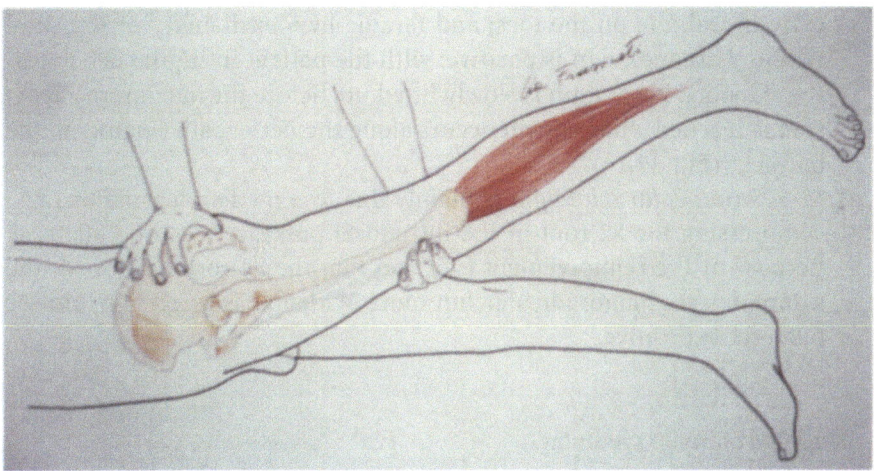

Fig. 12.13. Wassermann sign: hyperextension of the lower limb at the hip with knee extended

extension of the foot and of difficulty of walking on the heels. Faradic hypoexcitability of the long extensor muscle of the big toe, extensor digitorum and extensor digitorum brevis is frequent; Wasserman's test is positive (Fig. 12.13).

2) In *L5-S1 biradicular sciatalgia*, the S1 root is compressed on the intradural tract. This syndrome is rarer than the previous, and it is mainly due to median herniation. Therefore it is often bilateral. Pain irradiates along the posterior surface of the thigh, up to the poples and both antero-external surfaces of the leg, the back of the foot and the posterior surfaces of the leg. We can find: hypoesthesic zones in the corresponding areas, Achilles hyporeflexia, rare are flexia, hypotrophy of the triceps surae muscles, sometimes a difficulty in walking on the toes, and faradic hypoexcitability of the anterior and posterior muscles of the leg.

L5-S1 disk herniation. The V lumbar disk herniation follows, in order of frequency, that of the IV disk, causing two syndromes :

1) *S1 monoradicular syndrome* is the most common sciatalgia after the L5 monoradicular sciatalgia and it is mainly due to a lateral herniation. We can observe pain along the thigh and posterior surface of the leg, rare hypoesthesia on the posterior surface of the leg; Achilles areflexia, hyporeflexia, hypotrophy of the triceps surae muscles; sometimes diffi-

culty in walking on the toes; and faradic hypoexcitability of the sural triceps. Lasegue's sign is positive: with the patient in supine decubitus, the extended lower limb is slowly lifted up; before the maximum excursion is reached, intense pain occurs along the nerve path (mainly in the buttock) (Fig. 12.14).

2) *S1-S2 biradicular sciatalgia* is mainly due to a median herniation, also compressing the S2 root in the intradural passage. It can be bilateral. Because of the reinforcement function that the S2 root has for S1, the symptoms are monoradicular, but more evident. Lasegue's sign, uni- or bilateral, is positive.

Associated radicular syndromes

They are due to double herniation (quite rare) of the fourth and fifth disks, or of the third (or second) and fourth disks.

The clinical pictures are similar to that of L5-S1 biradicular sciatalgia

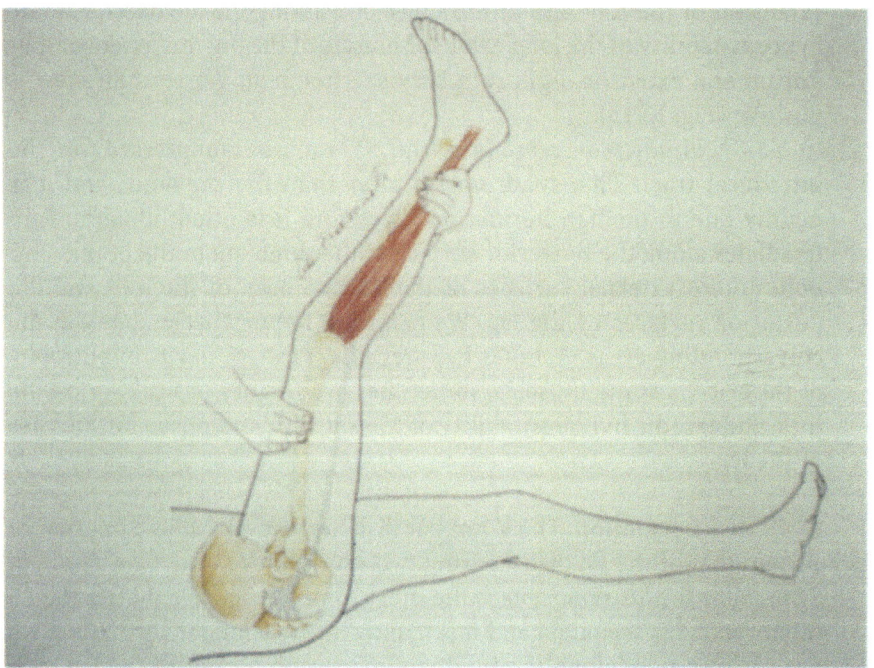

Fig. 12.14. Lasegue's sign: raising of the lower limb with knee extended and dorsal flexion of the foot

and L4-L5 biradicular cruro-sciatalgia, respectively, but with a different evolution and deficit grade. The symptoms are in relation to the root which has beeen compressed the longer by the herniated disk, or they are due to a single herniation having a transverse or vertical development and causing the simultaneous compression of two roots.

Cauda equina syndrome

This is a rare syndrome caused by lumbar disk herniation. It is often due to dorsomedian herniation. The clinical syndrome is various and polymorphous according to the disk involved, number of roots affected, and their grade of suffering. It is difficult to classify this syndrome, but didactically it is described by the following clinical varieties: complete lumbosacral from L2 to S5; incomplete lumbosacral from L3 to S5, from L4 to S5, from L5 to S5; inferior sacral S3-S4-S5. The motor disorders predominate and appear as paraparesis or flaccid paraplegia, occuring in the course of the first painful crisis. They can decrease progressively or, more rarely, abruptly. In rare cases, hypereflexia, Babinski and medullary sensory disorders are observed. Three factors determine the motor disorders, although in different measures according to the case: a mechanical factor, a dynamic factor (abrupt herniation protrusion and its mobility) and a vascular factor (simultaneous compression of one radicular or more radicular-medullary arteries).

Claudicatio intermittens caused by hernia

It is a rare syndrome caused by lumbar herniation, mainly at L3-L5 level. It is preceded by tenacious sciatalgic pain or dysesthetic-paresthetic disturbances. It appears after prolonged walking and can associate with a decrease in strength of the lower limbs with pyramidal signs; after a short rest the neurological examination is negative; the lumbar puncture can reveal an albuminocytologic dissociation. This syndrome is in relation to a transient medullary ischemia and not to direct compression (considering the level of the herniated disk). In fact, it is due to a compression of one or more radicular arteries serving the lumbar spinal cord when the anterior spinal artery is able to accomodate the higher metabolic demand during prolonged walking.

Acute paraplegia by lumbar hernia

It is a rare condition, preceded or accompanied by lumbar and lower limbs pains, by flaccid complete acute paraplegia with serious sphincteric disturbances, often associated with complete anesthesia of the lower limbs. We hypothesize a transient acute medullary ischemia due to involvement of the magna radicular artery, caused by the herniation or global injury of the radicular arteries which are satellite to the caudal roots.

The rachis lumbosacral plain X-ray can be normal or show narrowing of the involved diskal space and disappearance or decrease of lumbar lordosis. Caudography shows compression on the radicular pockets or dural sac (Fig. 12.15a,b). CT shows the herniation as a hyperdense image, median or lateral, extending into the conjugate foramina (intraforaminal herniation). NMR shows the herniation as a hypo-isointense area on T1-weighted images and a hypointense lesion on T2-weighted images (Figs. 12.16; 12.17).

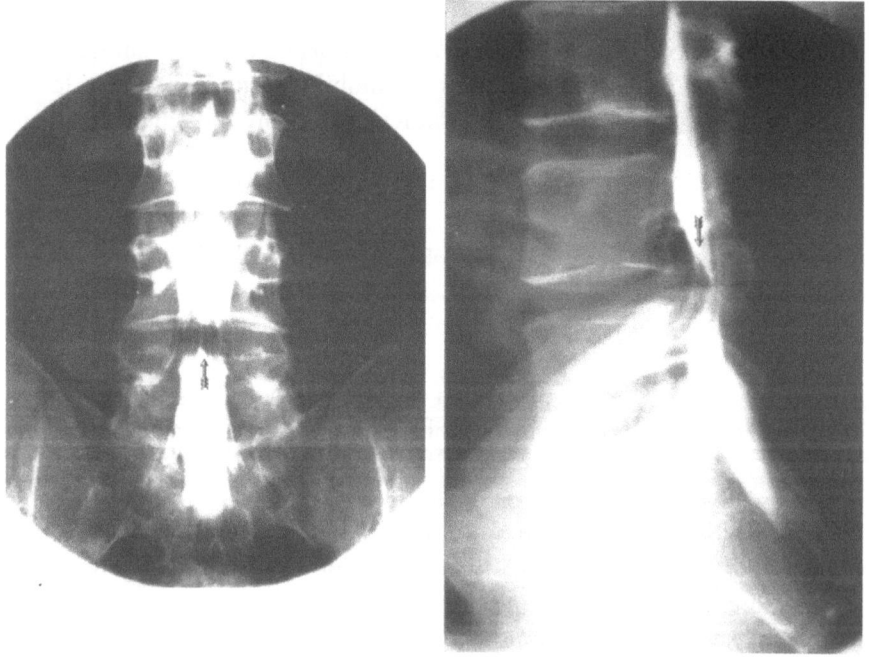

a   b

Fig. 12.15a,b. Disk herniation. Caudography. Compression on the dural sac at level of the L4-L5 intersomatic space with contrast medium block and not recognizable radicular pockets

Fig. 12.16. Left intra-extraforaminal lumbar herniation. NMR, axial view, T2-weighted image: circumscribed nucleus of tissue with diskal signal at L3-L4 with root compression

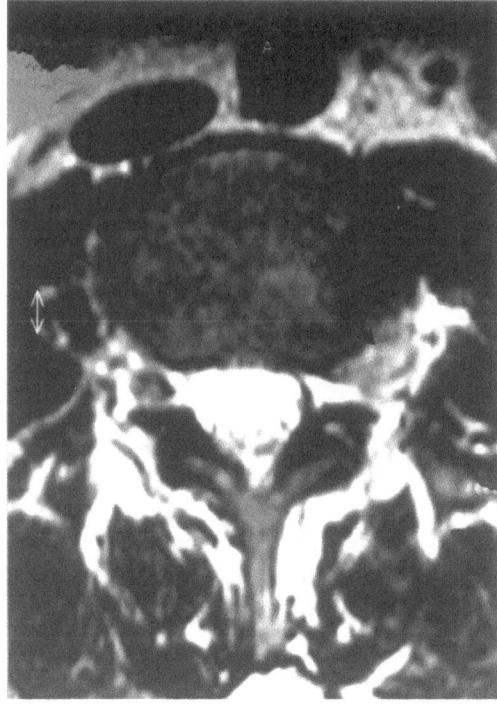

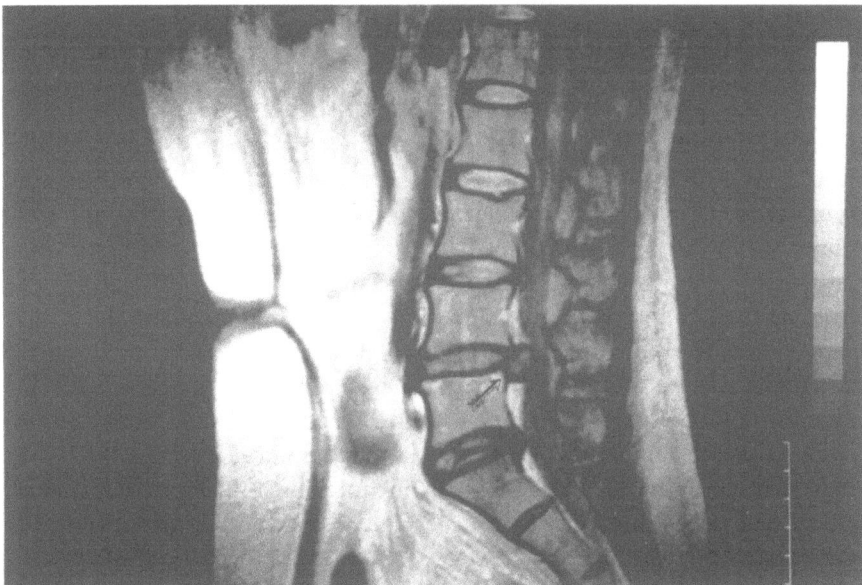

Fig. 12.17. Lumbar disk herniation. NMR, sagital view, T1-weighted image. Large disk herniation at L4-L5 with dural sac compression

The initial treatment is medical: rest for a few days and administration of cortisone, anti-inflammatory agents and muscle relaxants. Improvement can be achieved until complete regression of the pain. When the herniation is conspicous or excluded and the pain is intense and does not improve with therapy, surgical operation is necessary. It can be done by posterior microsurgery or percutaneous chemonucleolysis (introduction of a proteolytic enzyme, kimopapain, in the vertebral disk with lytic action on the nucleus pulposus). Sometimes, this procedure exposes to the risk of arachnoiditis due to the diffusion of the kimopapain in the rachis. The operation can also be done by nucleoaspiration with the optic fibers fibroscope.

Cervical spondylosis myelopathy

Cervical spondylosis is a secondary disease of chronic degenerative alterations of the intervertebral disks. It can flatten the intervertebral spaces and cause herniations, fissurations of the fibrous ring, and formation of marginal osteophytes.

This degenerative alteration occurs in a high percentage of people of middle (60%-75%) and advanced (95%) age (over 70 years). In a smaller number of cases, this lesion causes root or spinal cord damage with clinical signs of stress of the central or peripheral motor tracts, often intermingled to cause a polymorphous symptomatology. Nevertheless, the clinical picture reveals a clear cervical spinal cord stress. A slowly progressive spastic paraparesis, mixed signs in the upper limbs of central or peripheral motor tract involvement, and radicular and slight cordonal deficit are revealing symptoms of cervical spondylosis, especially if the pseudomyotonic phenomenon of the hand is present. This sign is characteristic of the disease (efficient and ready closure of the hand to fist followed by difficulty in the opening movement; pyramidal signs to the hand). Plain films (Fig. 12.18a) show one or more flattened intervertebral spaces with osteophytes which, in lateral projection, appear as osseous beaks reducing the anteroposterior diameter of the spinal canal to 4-5 mm. Dynamic X-rays show a more reduced or absent mobility of the flattened intervertebral spaces and increased mobility in the superior or inferior intervertebral spaces, changes of the conjugate foramina due to the osteophyte presence and increased lordosis.

CT shows an evident deformation of the posterior vertebral profile with irregular osteophytes marking the anterior profile of the dural sac. It also shows narrowing or obliteration of the conjugate foramina.

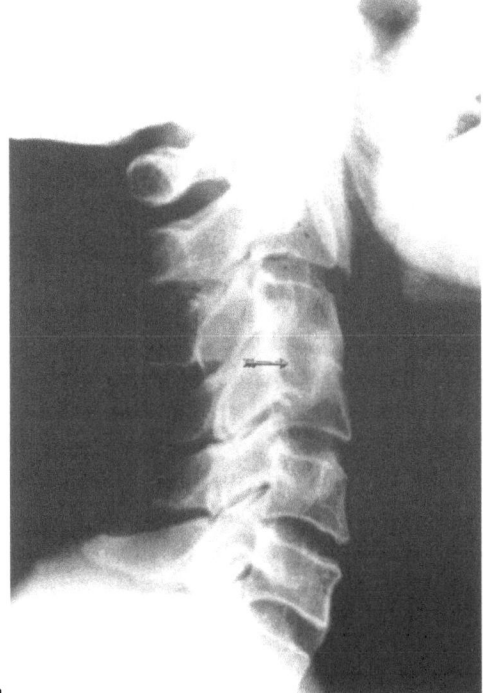

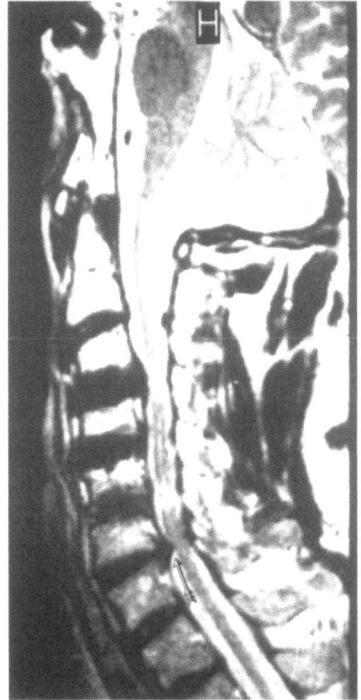

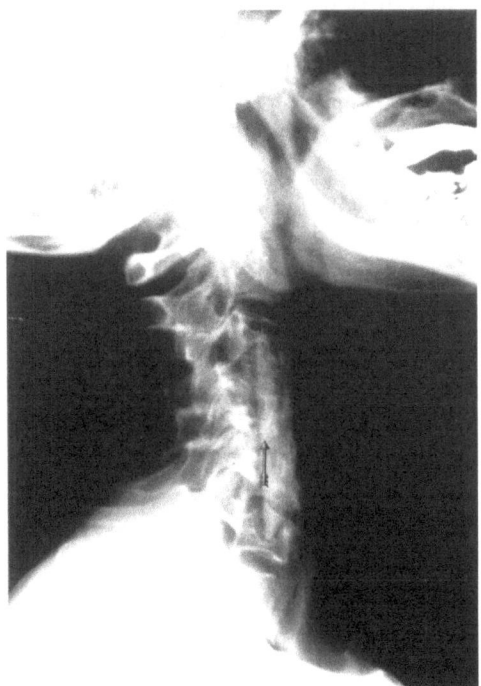

Fig. 12.18a-c. Cervical spondylosis. Cervical X-ray, lateral view (**a**): decrease of the C3-C4 interspace and reactive osteophytes. NMR cervical (**b**), sagittal view, T2-weighted image: anterior spinal compression at C6-C7 level. Cervical somatotomy (**c**). Cervical X-ray, lateral view: bone graft from the fibula

NMR shows, on T1-weighted images, alterations caused by the deformation of the vertebral canal and the medullary ischemic areas.

Therapy can be conservative or surgical. A nonoperative treatment is reccomended when the clinical picture is dominated by pain. The therapy should be based on anti-inflammatory and analgesic drug administration (steroids and NSAIDs). In resistant cases, the use of cervical collar or cervical traction is indicated.

Surgical therapy is indicated in patients with persistent pain and neurological deficit, especially if progressive (Fig. 12.18c). The operative procedure is based on the decompression of the spinal cord and nerve roots. The approach can be anterior, with the empityng of the intervertebral space, removal of the osteophytes by drill and curettes, and fusion of the vertebral bodies by bone graft. A median corpectomy and bone graft of iliac crest, fibula or titanium cages can be performed if more than three vertebral bodies are involved. A laminectomy can be associated if the spinal cord compression is due to yellow ligaments or spinal stenosis.

Lumbar stenosis

Lumbar spinal stenosis is characterized by reduction of the sagittal diameter of the spinal canal to less than 12 mm, with stenosis of the lateral recesses and intervertebral foramina. The stenosis can be mono- or plurisegmental and can involve part of the spinal canal or its entirety. The stenosis is classified into:
- Primary stenosis: congenital or developmental.
- Secondary stenosis: degenerative, post-traumatic, postinfective, iatrogenic, or caused by osteopathy.

Congenital stenosis is due to vertebral body or posterior arch congenital malformations. Among the developmental stenoses, achondroplasia is characterized by an early knitting fusion of the neurocentral synchondrosis with increased formation of periosteum and consequent laminae thickening, peduncles, and facet joint hypertrophy and with decreased spinal canal sagittal diameter. Achondroplasia is often associated with cervical and lumbar canal stenosis.

In secondary stenosis, the nervous structures are compressed by one or more conditions, such as a vertebral body or joint spondylolisthetic reactions, with or without spondylolisthesis.

Clinical picture

Women are more affected by degenerative stenosis, while congenital stenosis predominates in men. The most involved vertebral segments are L4-L5 and L3-L4. The symptomatology occurs in the fifth to sixth decades of life, when spondyloarthosis and degenerative disk disorders contribute to decrease an already congenitally reduced spinal canal.

The first symptom is pain, generally caused by trauma or other stress. Pain is diffuse, dysesthesic, lumbar, mono- and/or pluriradicular, and increases during walking or standing. The patient tends to walk with the trunk in flexion to reduce the pain. This is because trunk extension increases canal stenosis by bulging the ligamentum flavum and intervertebral disks into the spinal canal. Pain is more intense when the stenosis is associated with disk herniation. Claudicatio spinalis is another common sign. This is characterized by bilateral pain, dysesthesias (burning, cramps and cold sensations), and weakness of the legs. The spinal range of motion may be decreased. These signs appear and increase during walking or standing. This is due to nervous structure compression which blocks the vasodilation increasing blood circulation. The differential diagnosis should be made with ischemic vasculopathy of the lower limbs.

Radiological diagnosis

The anteroposterior radiography shows short laminae with sagittal direction and hypertrophic apophysis. In the lateral projections, a decreased length of the peduncles appears and a marked concavity of the joint facets is present, with osteophytes in the posterior edges of the vertebral bodies. The intervertebral foramina are decreased in the sagittal direction, due to a decrease in height of the intervertebral disk. The interpeduncular distance and the median sagittal diameter are decreased.

Sacculoradiography shows a generalized or segmental narrowing of the dural sac, an anterior, lateral, posterior dural impression, deformation in form of clepsydra, dyshomogeneous contrast medium distribution and periradicular sheath alterations (Fig. 12.19).

CT allows measurement of the median sagittal diameter: if less than 12 mm stenosis is present. CT also shows the foraminal stenosis, posterior bulging disk, posterior osteophytes, hypertrophy of the ligamentum flavum and morphological alterations of the dural sac (Fig. 12.20). NMR is the best diagnostic test, showing dural sac narrowing and the causes of the compression. The sagittal views provide diagnostic information similar to

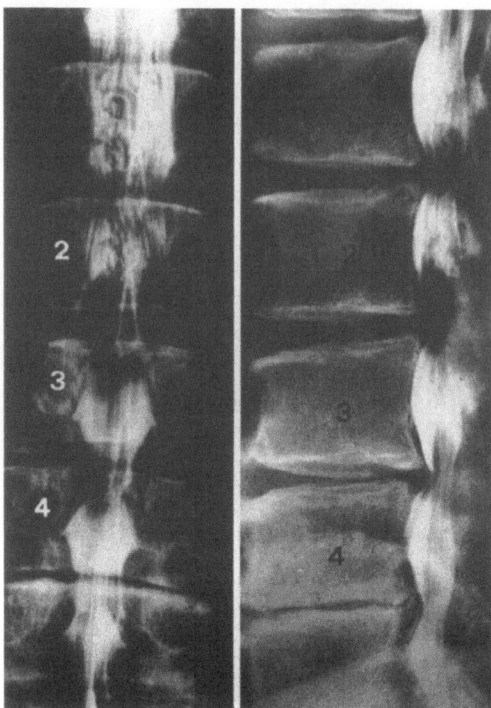

Fig. 12.19. Lumbar canal stenosis: myelography. Multiple compressions on the ventral portion of the dural sac with interruption of the contrast column at L1-L2 and L2-L3

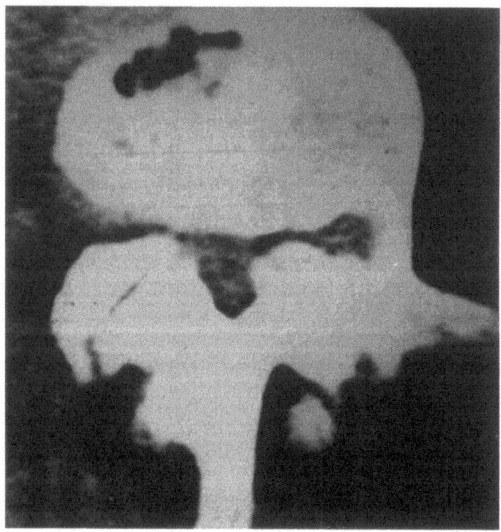

Fig. 12.20. Lumbar canal stenosis. CT of L4 vertebral body, axial view. Marked narrowing of the spinal canal due to joint facet hypertrophy and posterior ostheophytes

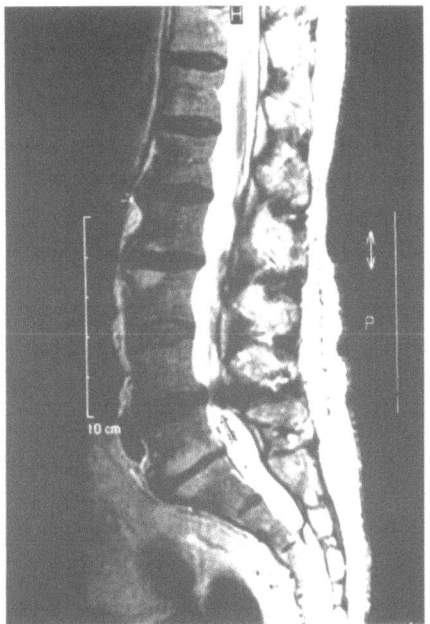 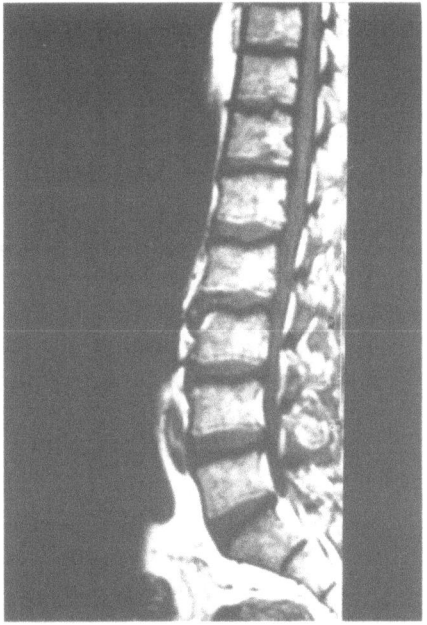

Fig. 12.21. Lumbar canal stenosis. MRI, sagittal view, T2-weighted image. Presence of marked segmentary stenosis at L4-L5 due to posterior osteophytes and yellow ligament hypertrophy

Fig. 12.22. Lumbar canal stenosis. MRI, sagital view, T1-weighted image. Severe narrowing of the anteroposterior diameter of the spinal canal with dural sac compression

sacculoradiography, but NMR can resolve if the compression is due to a disk herniation or a stenosis (Figs. 12.21; 12.22).

Therapy

The treatment can be conservative, based on physiotherapy and drug therapy (NSAIDs, steroids). Surgical therapy is indicated when there are neurological deficits (motor deficits or sphincteral disorders), and severe radicular symptoms not sensitive to a conservative treatment (pain, paresthesias). Surgical therapy is based on nervous structures decompression by laminectomy and facectomy (preserving the interarticular portion) and foraminotomy. The extension of the decompression depends on CT, NMR and myelography findings. These examinations allow to determine the extension in length of the abnormalities decreasing the diameter spinal canal.

Lumbar spondylolisthesis

The term spondylolisthesis means anterior sliding of the vertebral body on the underlying vertebra. In 50% of cases, spondylolisthesis is associated with interruption of the isthmus (spondylolysis). The most involved site is the fifth vertebra followed by the fourth vertebra.

Wiltse classified spondylolisthesis and spondylolysis into 5 categories:
- *Type I or dysplastic*: due to congenital alterations of the sacrum articular apophysis and V lumbar vertebra inferior articular apophysis.
- *Type II or isthmic*: the lesion is localized in the interarticular portion and is characterized by an isthmic fracture.
- *Type III or degenerative*: found in subjects affected by chronic disk disease, often localized between L4 and L5.
- *Type IV or traumatic*: provoked by severe trauma and causing lesions of the posterior vertebral arch, preserving the isthmic portion.
- *Type V or pathological*: due to bone diseases, such as metabolic or neoplastic osteopathies.

Etiopathogenesis

The theory of a congenital nature of spondylolysis is the most supported. According to this theory, there is a congenital anatomical predisposition to isthmic interruption. The interarticularis fractures occur in subjects which undergo constant mechanical stress, most commonly at the lumbosacral junction (such as weight-lifters, gymnasts, rugby players). The sliding of the vertebra with spondylolysis causes interarticular lysis and collapse of the capsuloligamentous and muscular structures. Sometimes, the spondylolisthesis without spondylolysis can be due to a lengthening of the vertebral isthmus.

From an anatomopathological point of view, the site of the isthmic lysis is covered by dense, reactive and fibrous tissue. The vertebral sliding can be more or less severe, until vertebral ptosis. Meyerding classified the spondylolisthesis into 4 grades. The sacrum is divided into quarters and the slip grade is defined in relation to the projecton site of the posteroinferior edge of the L5 body (Fig. 12.23). The disk herniation is rarely localized in the sliding interspace, but often localized in the superior space. Radicular suffering can occur in severe sliding, due to the stretching and compression of the nervous structures at the level of the decreased conjugate foramens and spinal canal.

Fig. 12.23. Meyerding's classification. The S1 body is divided into quarters, the posteroinferior position of the L5 body defines the grade

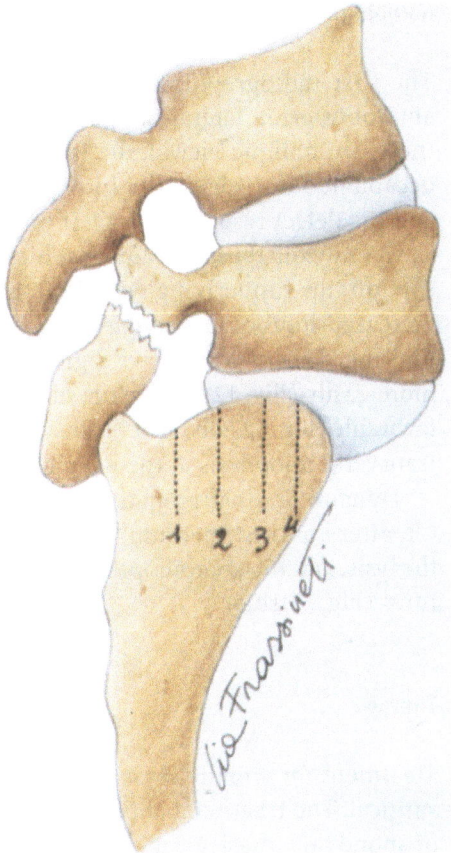

Clinical picture

Spondylolisthesis and spondylolysis rarely become symptomatic before adolescence or young adult age. Spondylolysis can appear with occasional lower back pain, usually occuring after prolonged standing or physical stress.

When spondylolisthesis occurs, lower back pain becomes more intense and frequent and can associate with radicular symptoms, until a cauda equina syndrome.

There are progressive postural changes: the center of gravity of the trunk is displaced forward with consequent hyperextension of the vertebral column, forward flexion of the pelvis (lumbosacral kyphosis), and dorso-abdominal circular cutaneous folds. At palpation, a step can be found among the spinous apophysis.

Radiological diagnosis

The first radiographic evaluation of the vertebral column must include anteroposterior, lateral-oblique and dynamic radiograms. In spondylolisthesis (in oblique views), the interruption of the isthmus appears as "the decapitated dog sign": the interarticular portion represents a dog's neck and the defect resembles a collar on the neck of the dog (Fig. 12.24).

Spondylolisthesis is radiographically characterized by a vertebral body slip on the underlying vertebral body (Fig. 12.25a), with or without increased lumbosacral angle or dome deformity of the sacrum superior limiting. This is a negative sign, because the sliding progression occurs more easily (Fig. 12.26a), while in case of an "S slip" the prognosis is more favorable (Fig. 12.26b). The "transverse sign" is due to an overlapping of the transverse apophysis at the wing of the sacrum (Fig. 12.27).

Dynamic radiography on lateral views, shows the vertebral body slip. CT, after contrast medium, and lumbosacral NMR allow the avalution of the lysis, and the anatomopathological state of the disk and radicular structures (Fig. 13.1b,c).

Therapy

Treatment for spondylolysis and spondylolisthesis can be conservative or surgical. The treatment choice depends on the clinical picture and the risk of spondylolisthesis progression. The risk factors are: 1) infantile or juvenile age, 2) gender (risk is greater in women), 3) dysplasia of the posterior

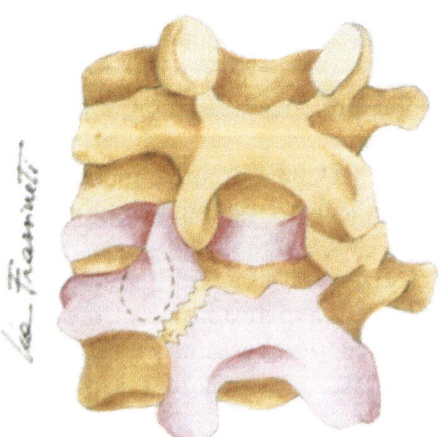

Fig. 12.24. Sign of the decapitated dog

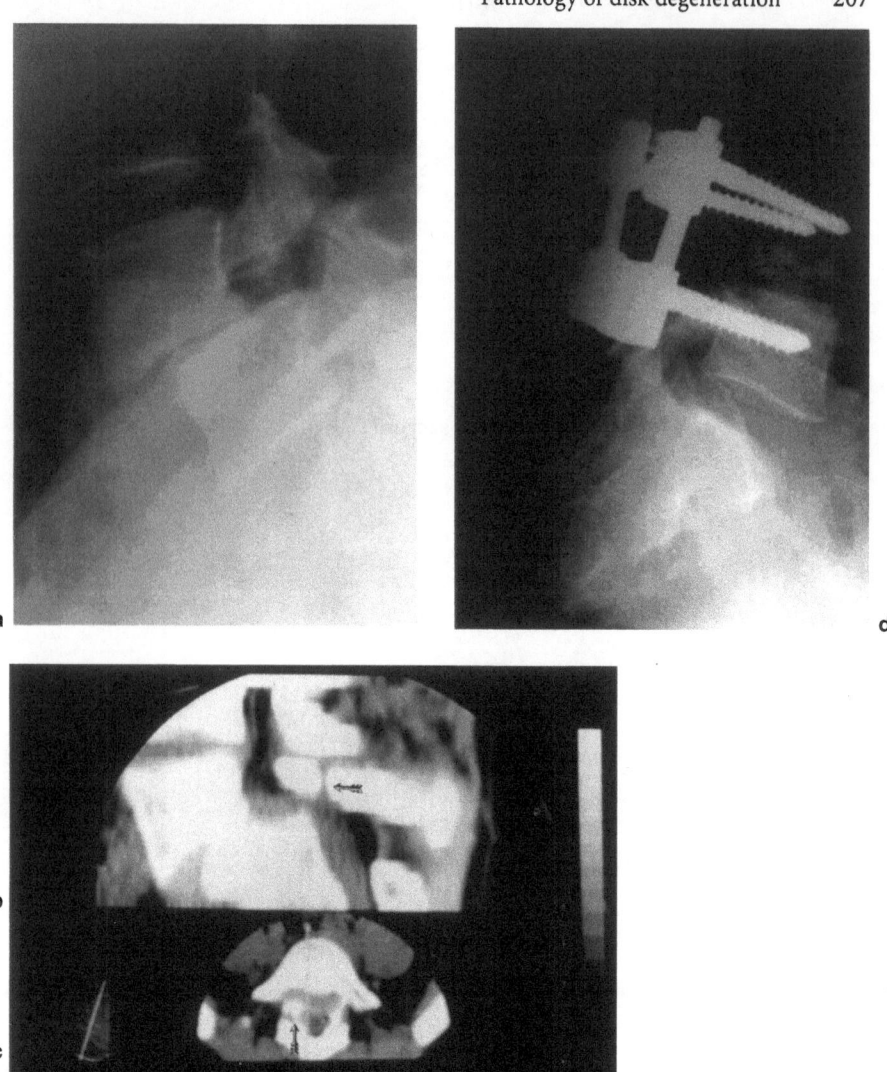

Fig. 12.25a-d. Spondylolisthesis of L5 on S1. Lumbar X-ray (**a**) and CT, sagittal view (**b**, **c**). Marked anterospondylolisthesis of L5 on S1 due to spondylolysis of L5. After surgical treatment with metallic plates and screws (**d**)

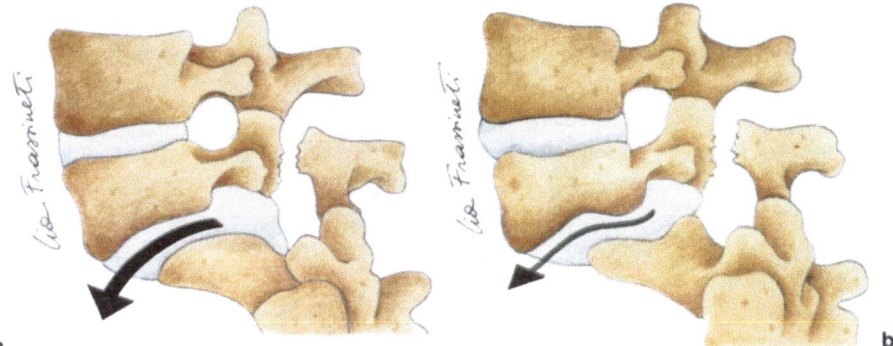

a   b

Fig. 12.26a,b. Dome sacrum (**a**) and (**b**) S sacrum sign

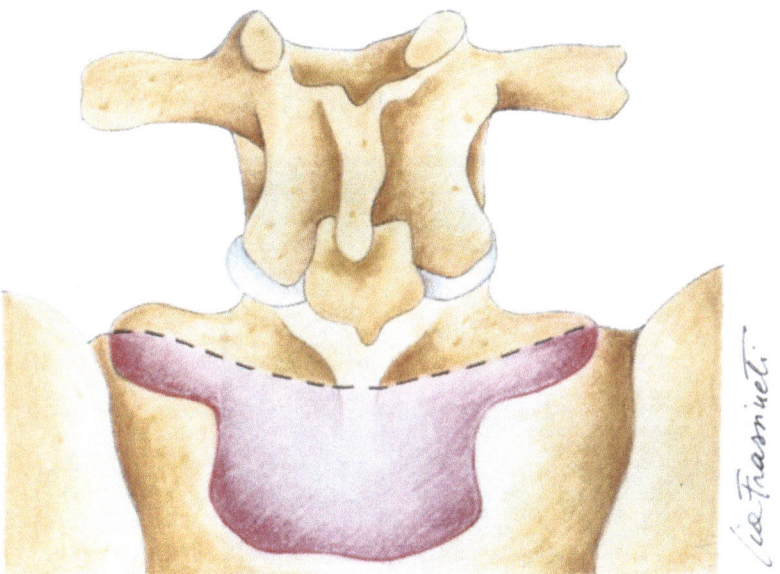

Fig. 12.27. Transverse or Pipino's sign

elements or spina bifida, 4) dome-like sacral surface, and 5) high slip angle. Conservative treatment is indicated in spondylolysis or spondylolisthesis of I grade. This treatment requires: analgesic and anti-inflammatory drugs and physiotherapy to strengthen the paravertebral musculoligamentous system, with or without dynamic orthopedic corsets.

Surgery is necessary after a conservative treatment failure and in patients with radicular symptoms and motor, sensory, or sphincteral deficits. The surgical procedure consists in anterior or posterolateral arthrodesis, with fusion by titanium plates, transpedicular screws and metalic cages to facilitate the alignment of the interspaces of the bodies (Fig. 12.25d). In patients with radicular symptoms, due to nerve structure compression at conjugate foramen level, a bilateral foraminotomy can be performed.

13. Peripheral nervous system diseases of surgical interest

Injuries to the peripheral nervous system that hold surgical interest are:
- traumatic and iatrogenic lesions,
- entrapment and canicular injuries, and
- tumoral injuries.

Traumatic and iatrogenic lesions

The causes of peripheral nervous system lesions are mechanical, termical, and electrical. Mechanical causes are the most frequent and they are provoked by sectioning, stretching, traction and compression.

Section lesions are caused by sharp objects, such as knives, glasses, lancets, and bony chips. The section can be total or partial, longitudinal or transverse. Usually, it is clean. In lesions associated with contusion and laceration, as in case of a lesion caused by a fluctuating saw, contusion, laceration and nerve substance loss can result.

Stretching and traction lesions are commonly associated with fractures, with or without luxation, and also occur during surgical divarication. They mantain the continuity of the nerve, although sometimes the force is sufficient to cause its rupture. This mechanism often causes brachial plexus lesions (delivery trauma, motorcycle accident, shoulder fracture-luxation), radial nerve lesions (fracture of humerus), and peroneal nerve lesions (shin bone and knee fracture-luxation).

Compression injuries damage a nerve by decreasing the blood flow or by a direct mechanical distortion. The severity of the lesion is related to the duration and intensity of the compression. Examples of compression lesions are: "saturday night paralysis", due to radial nerve compression in a drunk patient who tends to maintain an obliged position for a long time; lesions due to a wrong application of plaster, and fractures associated with considerable satellite hematomas.

A particular traumatic lesion is caused by intramuscular injection of pharmacologic substances. The mechanisms of damage can include neurotoxic action of the drug, direct damage of the needle on fascicles, and compression and tardy constriction of the scar.

Thermic lesions rarely involve the peripheral nerves, but patients affected by burns can present tardy peripheral deficit in relation to cicatricial fibrosis, producing a tourniquet effect.

Electrical lesions damage peripheral nerves by direct action of the electric current or by connected thermal effects. The severity of these lesions is related to the intensity of the discharge and the contact time.

According to the severity of the damage, nerve lesions can be distinguished, from the anatomofunctional point of view, into: neuroapraxia, axonotmesis, neurotmesis.

Neuroapraxia consists in a peripheral nerve functional loss, often incomplete and temporary. Its characteristic is the reversibility within hours or weeks, with the motor function often more affected than the sensory, without damage to the autonomic innervation. The most frequent cause is a light compression, traction or contusion of the nervous trunk.

The pathogenetic mechanism is connected to a localized biochemical disturbance, causing a conduction blockage or, if the compression is extended in time, a mechanism of segmental demyelinization.

The electrophysiological test (electromyography) shows, at the level of the functional lesion, a more or less complete blockage in conduction, while proximally and distally to the lesion itself the conduction is normal. Neuroapraxia does not require surgical treatment, due to the progressive and complete spontaneous recovery.

Axonotmesis is an immediate and complete loss of motor, sensory and autonomous functions distally to the nerve lesion. From an anatomical point of view, we can find a complete section of the axons and of the myelin sheath, with perineurium integrity. A distal wallerian degeneration and subsequent regeneration of the axon and of the myelin sheathe follow, with possible functional recovery of the nerve within a few months.

The most frequent causes of axonotmesis are fractures, lesions by compression, and injections.

Electromyography, at the level of the involved muscles at rest, does not show electric activity for 2-3 weeks, then fibrillation potentials begin to appear, progressively, followed by regeneration potentials.

Usually, the nerve has a spontaneous functional recovery within a few months; otherwise, surgical exploration is necessary.

Neurotmesis is a complete loss of motor, sensory and autonomic functions of the affected nervous trunk. Anatomically, we have complete section of the nerve or destruction of the nervous tissue for an extent in compatible with spontaneous recovery or, if there is an apparent macroscopic integrity, the cicatrization tissue causes a destruction of the structure which does not allow an anatomo-functional repair.

The most common causes of neurotmesis are: lacerations, tractions, serious crushes, direct lesions caused by bullets, and ischemic lesions.

The neurophysiological findings are similar to those of the axonotmesis.

Neurotmesis requires surgical treatment.

Therapy

It is useful to distinguish traumatic peripheral nervous lesions into open and closed, in order to give an indication for the surgical choice and the most suitable moment for the operation.

In open lesions, it is possible to check the morphological integrity of the nerve. When the nerve appears to be intact, the surgical procedure is not advisable, while it is necessary to suture the stumps if a partial or total section of the nerve occurred.

In closed lesions caused by traction, stretching, or compression, an early surgical operation is not advisable since it is possible to have spontaneous functional recovery of the nerve within weeks or months.

If clinical and electrophysiological tests do not show signs of nerve recovery within three months, a surgical exploration is required. The surgical technique for the repair of injured peripheral nerves consists in termino-terminal epineurial and interfascicular suture, if the gap is no longer than 1-2 centimeters. Otherwise, an autologous graft is performed using functionally unimportant sensory nerves (e.g. sural nerve, medial cutaneous nerve of the arm) (Fig. 13.2).

Entrapment or canicular syndromes

The entrapment neuropathies are peripheral nerve disorders affecting the nerve segments passing through osteofibrous canals or narrow orifices, in case a discrepancy between the diameter of the nerve and the diameter of

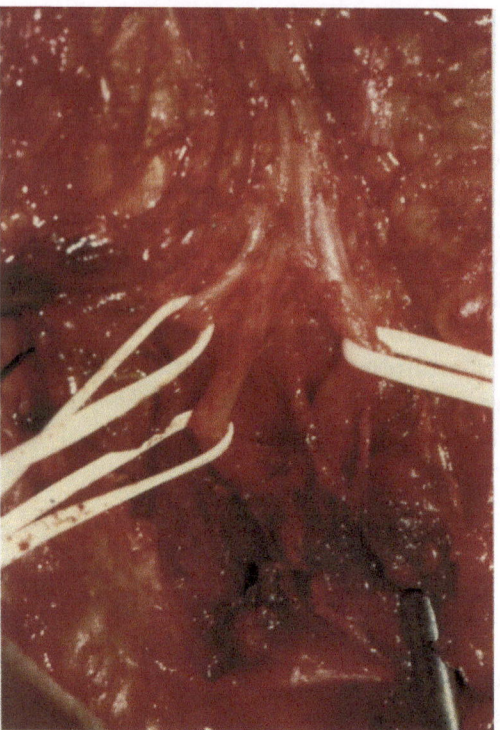

Fig. 13.1. External neurolysis surgical aspect of the common peroneal nerve

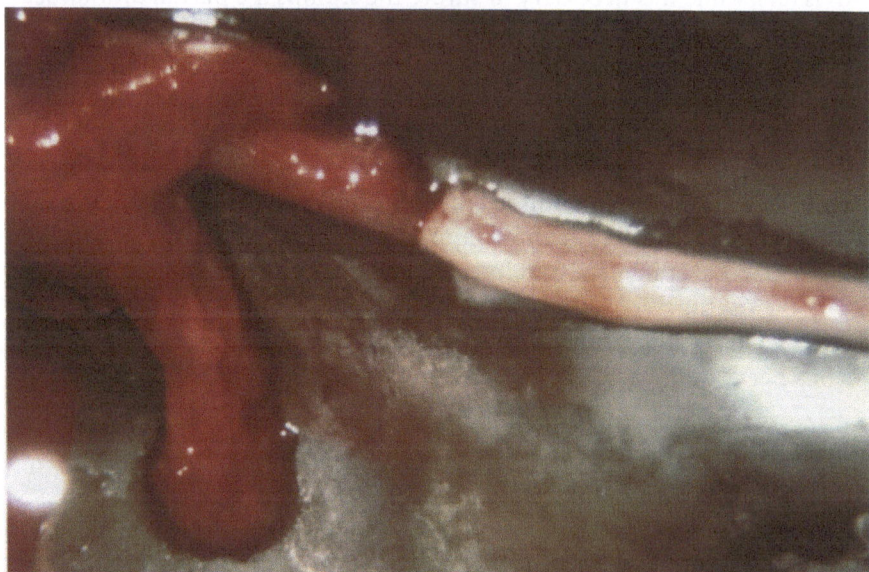

Fig. 13.2. Autograft surgical aspect of the median nerve with sural nerve

the osteofibrous canal is present. The reduction of the osteofibrotic tunnel can be caused by abnormal osseous projection, fractures, ligamentous hypertrophy, and inflammatory phenomena (tenosynovitis).

The nerve, in this anatomical constriction, undergoes direct mechanical compression and alterations of the intraneural vascular circulation with consequent hypoxia-anoxia and ischemia, responsible for functional and anatomical alterations. The severity of the damage is related to the grade of compression and to its duration.

Histologically, the big caliber myelinated fibers (motor and tactile sensitivity) of the chronically compressed peripheral nerve present alterations, while the unmyelinated dolorific fibers are scantly involved. Clinically, the neuropathy occurs with pain, paresthesias, sensory and motor deficiencies in the territory of distribution of the nerve affected by the constriction.

Classification of the canicular syndromes

Canicular syndromes of the upper limb

- Thoracic outlet or brachial plexus syndrome
- Suprascapular nerve syndrome
- Median nerve syndrome at lacertus fibrosus level
- Pronator syndrome
- Anterior interosseous nerve syndrome
- Posterior interosseous nerve syndrome or entrapment in Frohse's arch
- Ulnar nerve syndrome at elbow level
- Ulnar nerve syndrome at wrist level or Guyon's canal syndrome
- Carpal canal or median syndrome at wrist level

Canicular syndromes of the lower limb

- Syndrome by compression of the femoro-cutaneous nerve
- Syndrome by entrapment of the saphenous nerve
- Syndrome by compression of the common peroneal nerve
- Syndrome of the posterior nerve or tarsal tunnel syndrome
- Syndrome by compression of the digital collateral branches or Morton's syndrome

Thoracic outlet syndrome or brachial plexus syndrome

This is a very debated syndrome in terms of its pathogenesis, diagnosis and therapy. It is due to compression of the neurovascular group (brachial plexus, subclavian artery and subclavian vein) entering the thoracic outlet.

The thoracic outlet can be anatomically described as a triangle, in which the osseous component is formed by the vertebral column posteriorly, by the clavicle anteriorly, and by the first rib laterally. The muscular component is represented by the anterior and medial scalene muscles, which, with the first rib, form the triangle of the scalenes (Fig. 13.3).

Several causes are responsible for the narrowing of the costo-scalinic triangle: transverse mega-apophysis of C7, cervical rib, very high first thoracic rib with abnormal shape, hypertrophy and anomalous origin of the scalene muscles, and neurovascular fibers going through the scalene muscles fibers. The compression of the neurovascular group is possible in the interscalenic space, between the scalene muscles, between the clavicle and the first rib, and under the pectoral muscle.

Clinically, the thoracic outlet syndrome includes a neurogenic component and a vascular component. The neurogenic component is characterized by gnawing or pulsating pain in the suprascapular region, with dysesthesias that irradiate to the arm in the ulnar territory. The pain is increased by movement, limb tiredness, head rotation towards the healthy side and compression of the anterior scalene muscle.

The vascular syndrome, caused by subclavian artery compression or by reflected vasoconstriction subsequent to irritation of sympathetic branches, is rare and consists in cyanosis, edema, decrease of cutaneous temperature, pallor, and pain, and it is exacerbated by arm tiredness.

The diagnosis is based both on the clinical picture (Adson and Allen maneuvre) and on neuroradiologic tests (plain film, CT, NMR, angiography) which show the osseous, muscular and vascular malformations at the level of the thoracic outlet.

The neurophysiological findings show a decrease in the motor conduction velocity at scapular and axillary levels, in relation to the distal segments of the ulnar nerve.

The differential diagnosis is done in relation to the peripheral neuropathology of the ulnar and median nerves, at wrist and elbow levels, cervical radiculopathies, scapulohumeral periarteritis and brachial plexus neuritis.

Therapy can be conservative: physiotherapeutical treatment to correct posture or to strengthen the musculature of the scapulo-humeral girdle, change in life style and work habits, and periodical infiltrations with novocaine in the anterior scalene muscle. In there is no improvement, the ther-

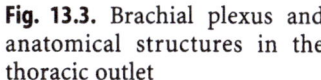 **Fig. 13.3.** Brachial plexus and anatomical structures in the thoracic outlet

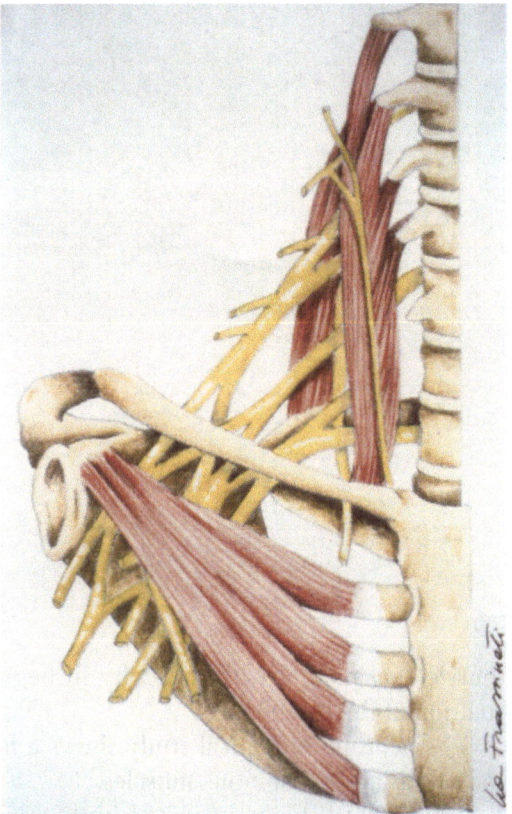

apy is surgical and consists in removing the causes responsible for the compression of the neurovascular group at the level of the thoracic outlet.

Suprascapular nerve syndrome

The suprascapular nerve is a mixed peripheral nerve, with a sensory component innervating the posterior part of the acromioscapular articular capsule and with a motor component innervating the supra- and subspinous muscles (abducting and revolving outwards the shoulder). It arises from the superior trunk (C5-C6) of the brachial plexus.

The syndrome is due to compression of the nerve on its route to the suprascapular foramen (Fig. 13.4). Clinically, during the initial or irritative stage, pain occurs in the posterior surface of the shoulder, with irradiation along the neck and the arm. The pain is aching, deep, and increases with shoulder movements. It can be associated with supra- and subspinous

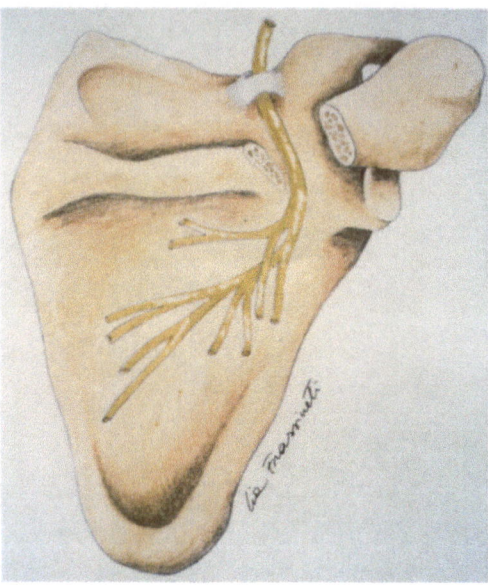

Fig. 13.4. Suprascapular nerve syndrome due to suprascapular foramen compression

muscle spasms and with difficulty in beginning outward abduction and rotation of the shoulder.

The neurophysiological study shows a neurogenic stress at the level of the supra- and subspinous muscles.

The surgical therapy consists in the section of the suprascapular ligament, if rest and therapy with anti-inflammatory agents (NSAID and steroids) are not successful.

Median nerve at lacertus fibrosus level syndrome

The median nerve is a peripheral nerve which originates from the medium trunk of the brachial plexus (C5-D1). Along the arm, it runs near the humeral artery; at the level of the elbow fold, it runs behind the bicipital aponeurosis (lacertus fibrous) and in front of the anterior brachial muscle; on its route to the forearm, it runs between the heads of the pronator muscle and under the ligament of the flexor digitorum superficialis muscle and, at the level of the forearm, in the deep aponeurosis of the flexor digitorum superficialis muscle.

The syndrome is caused by the fibrous thickening of the lacertus which compresses the median nerve during muscular contraction (Fig. 13.5).

The clinical picture, often unclear, is characterized by tenderness or diffuse pain in the forearm, by paresthesias in the territory of the median nerve at the level of the hand, especially of the index and wrist, and grasp weakness. Pain increases with forearm pronation movements, while a nocturnal increase, typical of the carpal tunnel syndrome, is not present.

Electromyography shows a muscular stress in the median nerve distribution territory, distally to the compression site.

The therapy, at first, is conservative (rest, administration of NSAID and steroids). In resistant cases, surgical therapy consists in the resection of the adherencies which compress the nerve.

Pronator syndrome

It is due to compression of the median nerve on its path between the two heads of the pronator and under the ligament of the musculus flexor digitorum superficialis. The most frequent causes are work activities involving forearm movements, especially forced pronation and supination (e.g. tennis, frequent use of screwdriver). Clinically, the patient feels diffuse

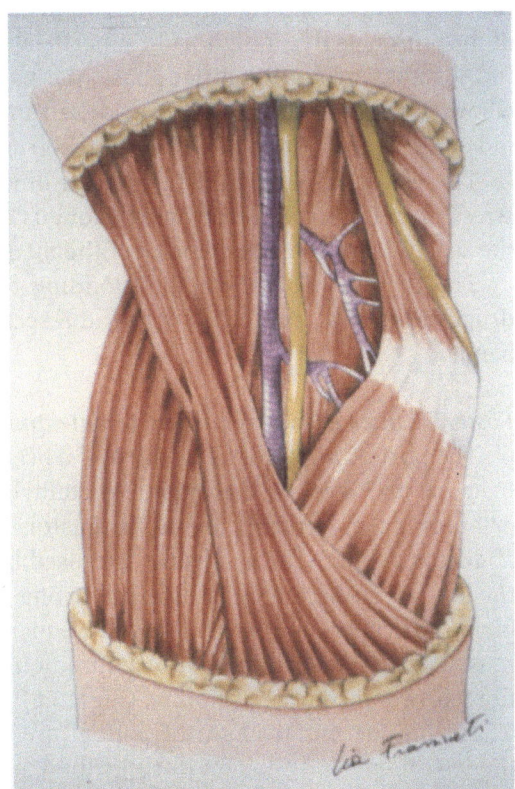

Fig. 13.5. Compression site of median nerve at the lacertus fibrous level

pain, which from the forearm spreads to the hand and increases by compression of the pronator muscle and by forced movements of pronation and supination. Hand paresthesias in the territory of the median nerve are also present.

The electrophysiological test (electromyography) shows a neurogenic stress in the muscular territory of distribution of the median nerve, without involvment of the pronator muscle.

The therapy, conservative at first, consists in a change in work habits, systemic administration of NSAID and steroids, and cortisone injections in the tendon of the round pronator muscle. In resistant cases, surgical therapy is recommended and it consists in the resection of the fibrous bands compressing the nerve.

Anterior interosseous nerve syndrome

This nerve arises from the median nerve at the level of the round pronator heads. It is mainly a motor nerve which innervates the musculi flexor pollicis longus, the flexor digitorum profundus and the pronator quadratus. The syndrome is due to compression of the nerve on the deep surface of the musculus flexor digitorum superficialis in the entrance foramen, into the sheath. During the initial phase, the patient feels a tenderness in the elbow and forearm, followed by a deficit in the flexion of the thumb and index distal phalanx and a deficit in the arm pronation.

The electrophysiological test (electromyography) shows a neurogenic stress of the musculi flexor pollicis longus and pronator quadratus, while the sensitive conduction velocity of the median nerve is normal.

The therapy, in cases not responding to rest and anti-inflammatory drugs, is surgical and consists in the resection of the nerve constriction bands.

Posterior interosseous syndrome or entrapment in Frohse's arch

The posterior interosseous nerve is a branch of the radial nerve. It originates at the level of the lateral epicondyle and innervates the musculi extensor carpi radialis brevis, supinator brevis, extensor pollicis and abductor pollicis. The syndrome is caused by the compression of nerve at the level of Frohse's arch (which is a strong fibrotendinous ring at the origin of musculus supinator brevis) subsequent to rheumatic sclerosis of the musculus supinator brevis. The syndrome may also result from traumatic fibrosis or intermuscular lipoma (Fig. 13.6).

During the initial stage, the patient presents tenderness at the level of the lateral epicondyle, pain during elbow movements, lack of strength in extension and abduction of the thumb, extension of the finger at

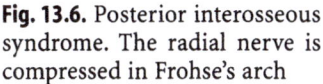
Fig. 13.6. Posterior interosseous syndrome. The radial nerve is compressed in Frohse's arch

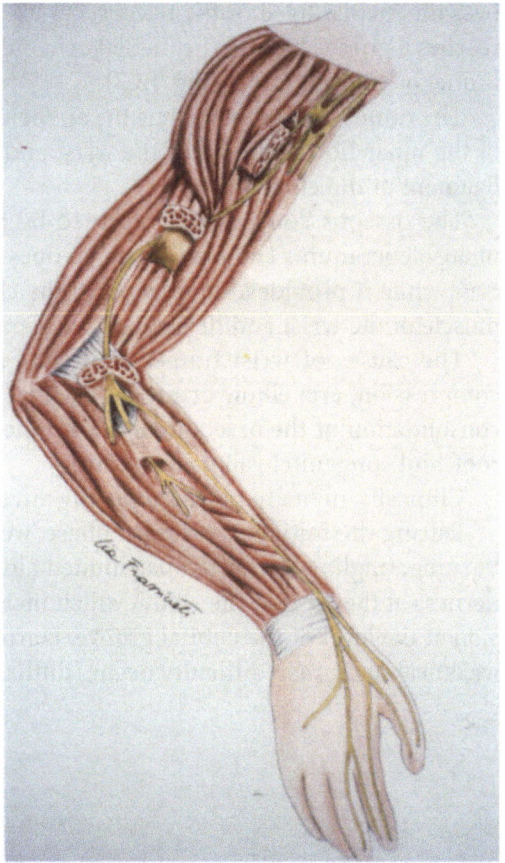

metacarpal and phalangeal articulations and wrist extension in radial deviation. There are no sensory disorders.

Electromyography shows neurogenic stress at the level of the muscles innervated by the posterior interosseous nerve, while the velocity of sensory conduction of the radial nerve is normal.

The therapy, at first, is conservative. It consists in rest and the administration of NSAID and steroids. In the absence of results, surgical therapy, consisting in the resection of Frohse's arch or of other constrictor fibrous bands, is indicated.

Ulnar syndrome at elbow level

The ulnar nerve arises from the medial cord of the brachial plexus (C8-D1). Along the arm, it crosses the humeral artery medially and it passes over the medial head of the triceps. On its passage through the forearm, it reaches a groove behind the medial epicondyle and crosses an osteofibrous tunnel or cubital tunnel (Fig. 13.7).

The tunnel roof is formed by the aponeurotic insertion of the two heads of the ulnar flexor muscle of the wrist and by the insertion of the medial ligament of the elbow joint.

The osseous component is formed by the medial epicondyle and the ulnar oleocranum. The median nerve does not contribute branches to the arm, while it provides innervation to the elbow joint and the ulnar flexor muscle of the wrist and flexor digitorum profundus musculus.

The causes of wrist tunnel reduction, and consequently of the ulnar compression, are: elbow arthrosis, fractures with vice of position or with consolidation of the osseous callus, acromegaly, rheumatic sclerosis of the roof, and congenital valgus dislocation.

Clinically, men are more frequently affected and it can be bilateral.

During the initial or irritative phase, we can observe paresthesias, as a burning, tingling sensation distribuited along the ulnar territory, and tenderness at the level of the elbow, which increases with the digital compression at the level of the cubital groove. During the slow or deficitary phase, weakness and grasp difficulty occur (difficulty in sewing, buttoning) relat-

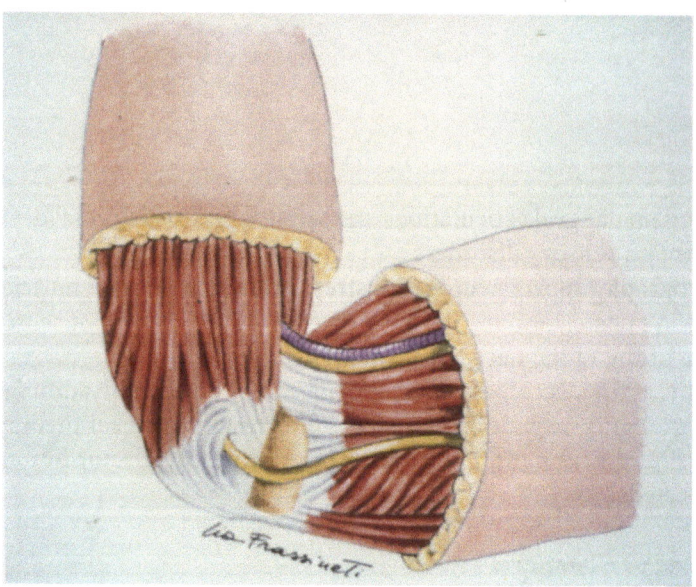

Fig. 13.7. Ulnar at elbow level compression site

ed to the deficit of the hand ulnar flexor muscle, of the interosseous, and of the thumb adductor muscle. During the physical test, a hypotenar eminence hypotrophy can be observed.

The electrophysiological test shows decreased conduction velocity of the ulnar nerve at the level of the elbow compared to the antibrachial tract.

The differential diagnosis can be done in relation to: C8 cervical radiculopathy by hernia of the disk, neurinomas, meningiomas, thoracic outlet syndrome, and Pancoast's syndrome. The therapy, during the irritative stage, consists in NSAID, cortisone and rest; if muscular atrophy and deficit occur, surgical therapy is urgently needed not to compromise the possibility of functional recovery. The surgical therapy consists in ulnar decompression and its transposition (Fig. 13.8).

Ulnar syndrome at wrist level or Guyon's canal syndrome

The ulnar nerve, at the transition between forearm and wrist, enters an osteofibrous canal (Guyon's recess or ulnar carpal tunnel) localized in the proximal part of the hypothenar eminence. The medial part of the osteofibrous canal is formed by the pyriform bone and the ulnar flexor tendon of

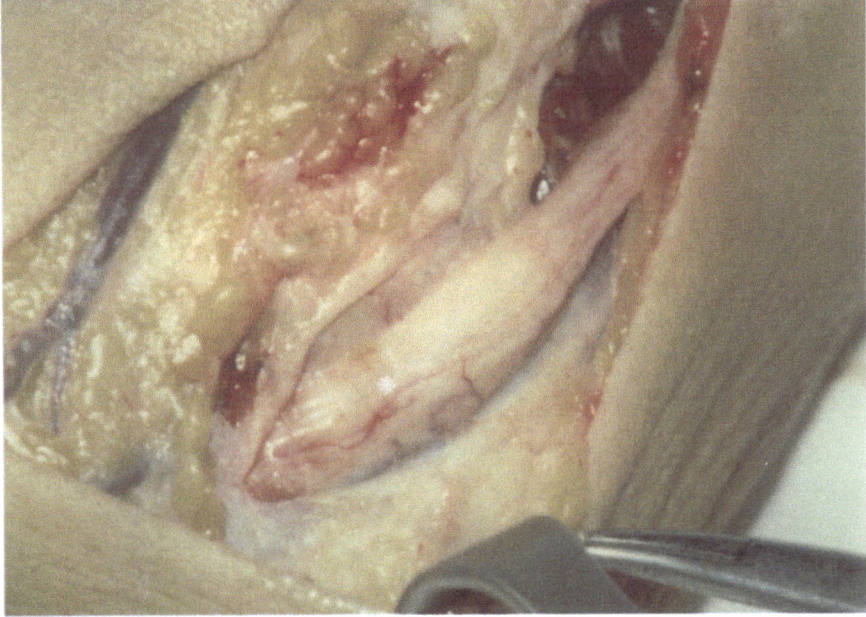

Fig. 13.8. Surgical aspect of ulnar nerve compression in the epitrochleo-oleocranic groove

the wrist; the lateral wall by the ulnar surface of the uncinate bone; the roof is delimited by the volar ligament of the wrist and of the small palmar muscle; the floor by the pyso-uncinate ligament and the reticulum of the flexors (Fig 13.9).

Causes of compression of the ulnar nerve in the carpal tunnel are: fractures of the uncinate process or of the pyriform, occupational microtraumas, rheumatic sclerosis of the canal, and tendinous cyst.

Clinically, during the initial or irritative phase, nocturnal paresthesias and hypoesthesias occur in the territory of ulnar distribution, increased by palpation at the level of the hypothenar eminence and of the hand. During the late or deficitary phase, the clinical picture is similar to that of the ulnar nerve syndrome at elbow level, but without forearm muscular deficit.

The electrodiagnostic test shows: normal motor conduction velocity of the ulnar nerve in the segment from the elbow to the thumb, increased latency distally to the abductor muscle of the little finger and first dorsal interosseous muscle, and decrease of the respective sensitivities.

Therapy is generally surgical and consists in the exploration of Guyon's canal region and in the elimination of the causes responsible for the nerve compression.

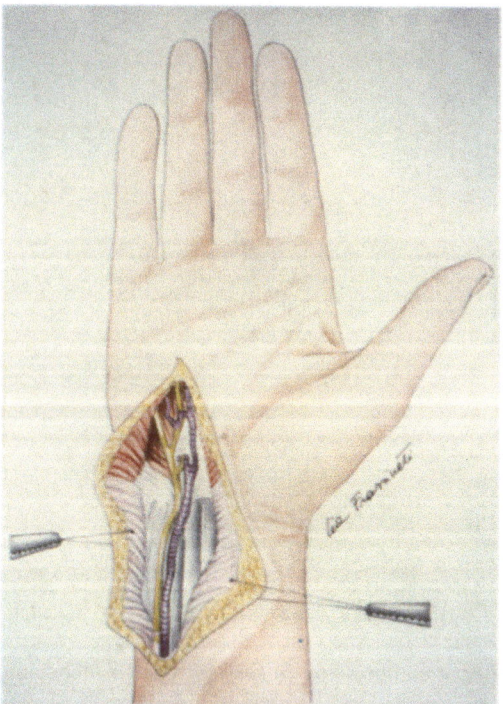

Fig. 13.9. Exposure of the ulnar nerve at wrist and hand level after volar ligament of the carpal and palmar aponeurosis incision

Carpal tunnel syndrome

The medial nerve, in its transition from the forearm to the wrist, crosses an osteofibrous canal, called carpal tunnel, localized in the proximal part of the thenar eminence. The carpal tunnel is composed, at a deep level, of an osseous component or carpal groove; at a superficial level by a strong transverse ligament which is in continuity, in the inferior part, with the palmar fascia and is inserted on the tubercle of the scaphoid and trapezium bones laterally, and on the pyriform and uncinate ones medially (Fig. 13.10).

This syndrome is due to a discrepancy between the canal volume and its contents. The causes are: thickening of the transverse ligament of the wrist, luxation of the wrist joint and incorrect fusion of the osseous callus after fracture of the carpal bones, and inflammatory processes such as tenosynovitis of the retinaculum of the flexors.

The symptomatology, during the initial or irritative phase, is characterized by paresthesias, in most cases nocturnal, a tingling or dead hand sensation which can evolve into pain with distribution on the thumb and on the first three fingers. The percussion of the wrist (Tinel's sign) causes paresthesias and pain along the distribution territory of the median nerve at the level of the hand.

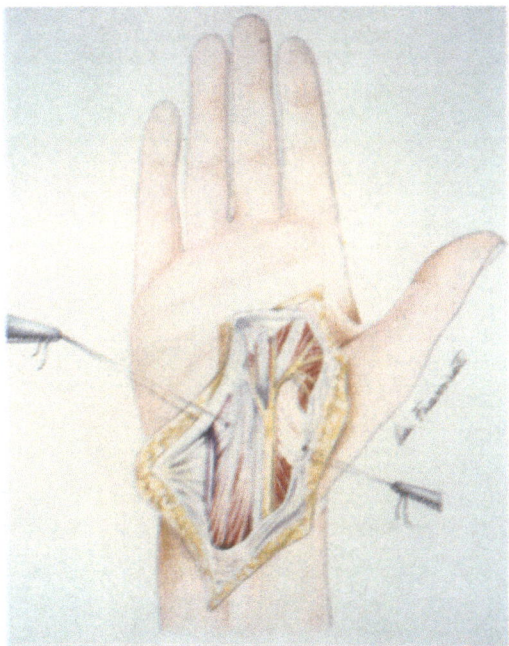

Fig. 13.10. Exposure of the median nerve at wrist and palm levels after transverse ligament incision

Fig. 13.11. Surgical aspect of median nerve debridement at wrist level

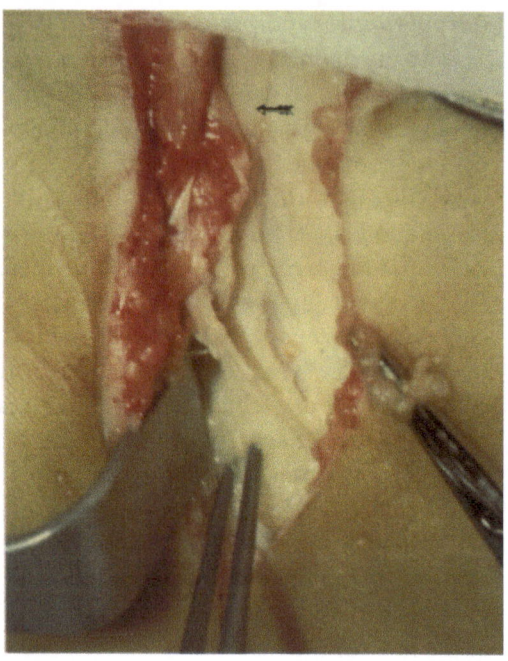

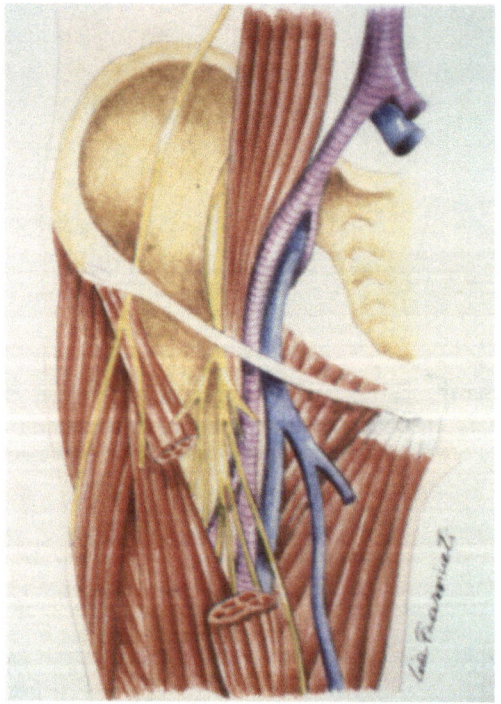

Fig. 13.12. Lateral cutaneous of the thigh nerve syndrome due to inguinal ligament compression

During the late or deficitary phase, motor deficit occurs, such as easy fatigue and difficulty in performing movements with the fingers, especially opposition of the thumb. Atrophy of the thenar eminence occurs as well.

The neurophysiological study shows a decrease of the sensitivity conduction velocity of the median nerve under the carpal tunnel. The differential diagnosis includes the compression of the median nerve at the level of the round pronator, with a C6-C7 radiculopathy, a thoracic outlet syndrome with cervical syringomyelia, and amyotrophic lateral sclerosis.

The therapy, during the initial stage when the symptomatology is limited to paresthesias and pain, consists in rest, NSAID, steroids and diuretics.

During the deficitary stage, operation is necessary to decompress the nerve. It consists in the section of the transverse ligament and in the exploration of the wrist floor to exclude hyperostotic phenomena and cystic formation (Fig. 13.11).

Lateral cutaneous nerve of the thigh compression syndrome

The cutaneous nerve of the thigh is a sensory nerve. It divides into two terminal branches, innervating the anterolateral surface of the thigh and the superolateral surface of the nates (Fig. 13.12).

Generally, the compression occurs at the level of the inguinal ligament. The main causes of the compression are: residual scarring due to past trauma, fascial sclerosis, and compression of the femoral artery or vein.

The symptoms are: pain, paresthesias, dysesthesias in the anterolateral surface of the thigh and hypoesthesia, increased by extension movements of the thigh.

The differential diagnosis is with the lumbosacral pain due to hernia of the disk compressing the L2 root, or with neoplastic lesions.

At first, the therapy is conservative (rest, NSAID and cortisone administration), but in drug resistance cases surgery becomes necessary to decompress the nerve.

Saphenous nerve entrapment syndrome

The saphenous nerve is exclusively sensory and represents the most important cutaneous branch of the femoral nerve. It arises under the inguinal ligament, enters Hunter's canal (or subsartorious canal or abductor canal), crosses it along the thigh in a lateromedial direction and, before reaching the knee, exits the canal at the level of the subsartorious roof, distributing its terminal branches on the medial surface of the leg.

The compression occurs at the level of the exit point from the subsartorious canal. Clinically, this syndrome manifests itself in an acute or insinuating way, with a violent and strong pain at the medial surface of the knee. The pain is increased by limb fatigue. This syndrome usually affects young people and women.

Palpation at the nerve emergence site (about 20 cm above the medial surface of the knee) causes or increases pain.

The differential diagnosis includes the L2-L3 diskal radiculopathy.

The initial therapy consists in rest, NSAID and steroid administration.

In resistant cases, the surgical decompression of the nerve is performed at the level of the subsartorious fascia in the emergence zone.

Common peroneal nerve syndrome

The common peroneal nerve is a terminal branch of the sciatic nerve. It arises at the level of the popliteal hollow and it is divided into two terminal branches: the superficial peroneal nerve and the deep peroneal nerve. It is a mixed nerve: the muscular component innervates the anterior tibial muscle and the extensor digitorum musculus used for foot dorsiflexion and the long peroneal muscle and short peroneal muscle used for foot abduction, while the sensory component innervates the skin of the mediolateral part of the leg and of the dorsal part of the foot.

The compression of the common peroneal nerve occurs at the level of the calf bone head, where the nerve is superficial, easily exposed to trauma and strictly fixed to the periosteal structures (Fig. 13.13).

The main causes responsible for nerve stress are: traumatic, like tearing or fractures of the peroneal head, or expansive lesions like osteomas, lipoma, neurofibromas, and tendinous cysts.

The clinical picture is characterized by progressive deficit in the dorsal flexion and abduction of the foot, responsible for a stepping gait with dropping of the foot. It is also characterized by hypo-anesthesia on the leg lateral region and foot dorsal region.

Electromyography shows a neurogenic stress limited to the muscles innervated by the common peroneal nerve.

The differential diagnosis includes the L5 radiculopathy, and is based on the presence or absence of low back pain or lumbosciatalgia and on the neurophysiological test findings.

The therapy is, generally, surgical and consists in the decompression of the common peroneal nerve.

Tarsal nerve syndrome or tibial nerve syndrome

The tarsal tunnel is an osteofibrous canal, localized in the posterior and inferior part of the medial malleolus. In its external part, it is delimited (roof of the tunnel) by the lancinatus ligament or the flexor retinaculum

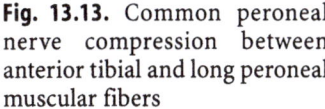

Fig. 13.13. Common peroneal nerve compression between anterior tibial and long peroneal muscular fibers

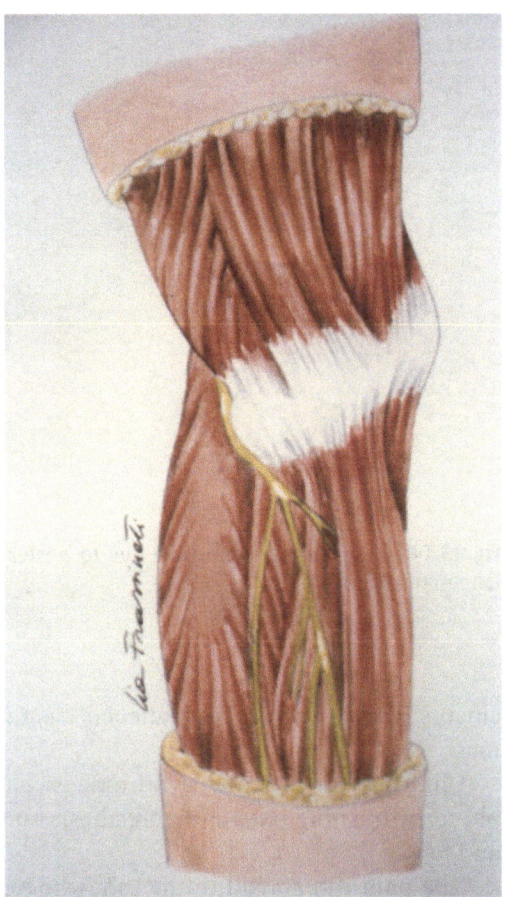

and by the osseous component (medial surface of the heel bone and posterior surface of the medial malleolus) (Fig. 13.14).

The posterior tibial nerve, and the homonymous vessels, go through the tarsal tunnel. The posterior tibial nerve, terminal branch of the sciatic nerve, navigates along the posterior surface of the leg, deeply to the soleus muscle and, after crossing the tarsal tunnel, it divides into two terminal branches: the medial and the lateral plantar nerves.

It is a mixed nerve: the motor component innervates the foot and toe intrinsic muscles, consolidating the toe abduction and adduction, while the sensory component innervates the skin of the foot tip, the external edge and the distal part of the toes.

The most frequent causes of posterior tibial nerve compression are: lan-

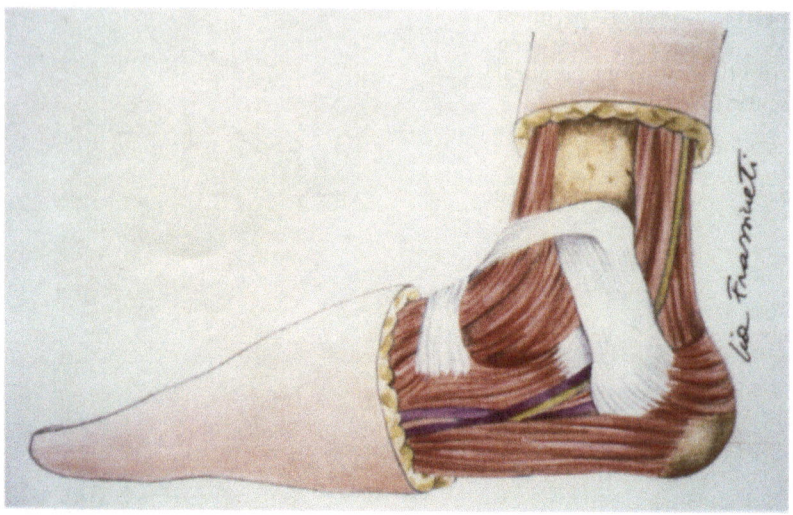

Fig. 13.14. Tarsal tunnel syndrome due to posterior tibial nerve compression under lancinatus ligament

cinatus ligament sclerosis, malleolar fractures, tendinous cyst, and neuromas.

Clinically, tarsal tunnel syndrome is characterized, during the irritative phase, by burning pain and paresthesias on the plantar surface of the foot and toes.

The pain can spread to the calf, while the heel bone is not necessarily involved. The pain decreases with rest, and increases with fatigue. Tinel's sign is positive on the retromalleolar groove.

During the deficitary phase, hypotrophy and atrophy of the foot intrinsic muscles and plantar hypoesthesia are associated with the previous symptoms.

The electrodiagnostic test shows a decrease in amplitude of the great toe abductor muscle and toe quadrate muscle evoked potentials.

Prolonged motor latency in the abductor of the little toe and the big toe can be observed as well.

The treatment is surgical and consists in the decompression of the posterior tibial nerve at the level of the osteofibrous tunnel and in the section of the lancinatus ligament and the deep fibrous bands strangling the nerve.

Collateral digital branches compression syndrome or Morton's disease
This syndrome is caused by an entrapment of the canals digital nervous branches between plantar aponeurosis, deep aponeurotic fascia and metatarsal heads (Figs. 13.15; 13.16).

The most frequent causes are the metatarsophalangeal arthrosis, thickening and sclerosis of the plantar aponeurosis, neromas, and tendinous cyst.

The syndrome is characterized by pain and paresthesias at the level of the forefoot and toes.

Tinel's sign is positive. Interdigital hypoanesthesia can be observed at a physical examination.

During the first phase, the therapy consists in administration of NSAID and corrective supports. In case of persistence of symptoms, surgical treatment is necessary. It consists in the isolation and resection of the compressed digital branch.

Tumoral lesions

Tumors of the peripheral nerves constitute a relatively rare pathology. In relation to their biological characteristics, tumors of the cranial and spinal nerves are classified into:

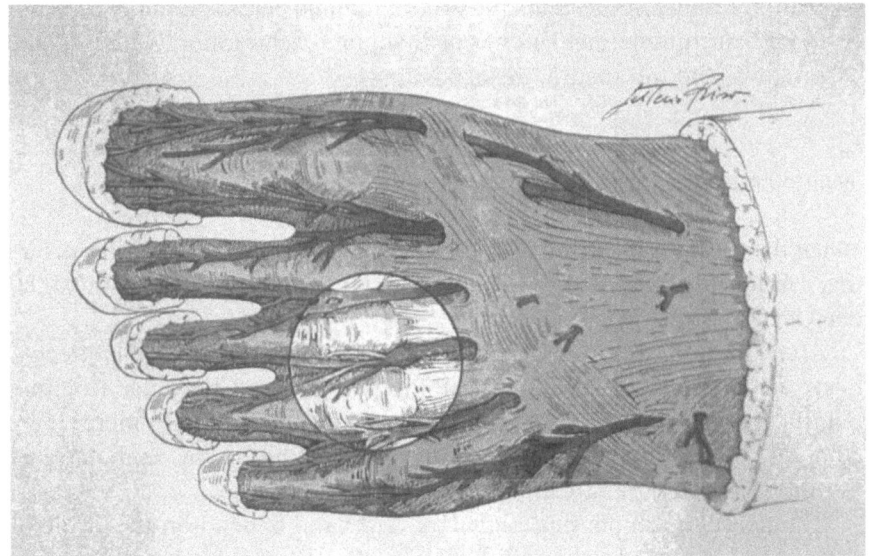

Fig. 13.15. Anatomical diagram of Morton' s neurinoma

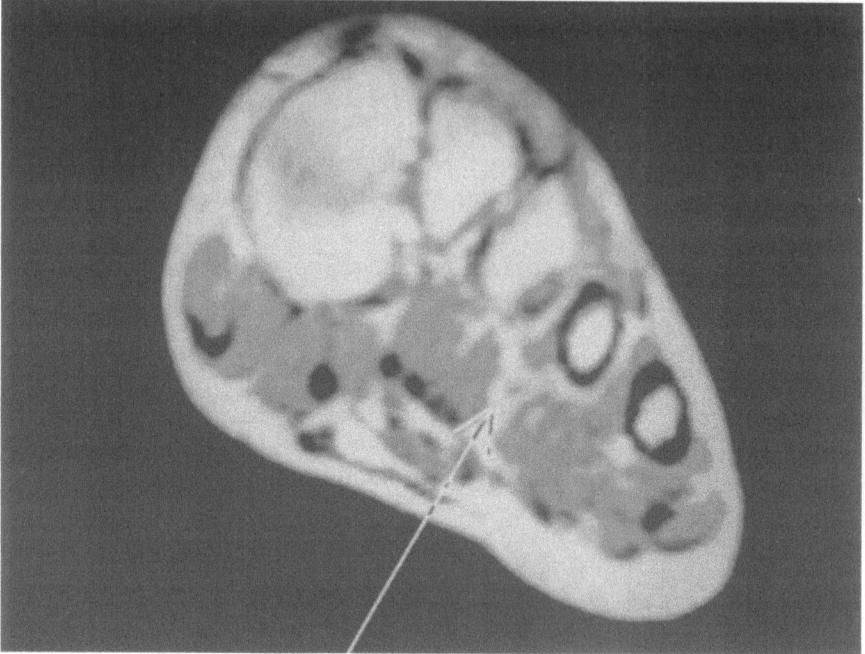

Fig. 13.16. Foot NMR: Morton's neurinoma

- Benign tumors of ectodermic origin: neurinoma, neurofibroma.
- Benign tumors of mesodermic origin: lipoma, hemangioma.
- Malignant tumors: neurinoma or malignant schwannoma, neurogenic sarcoma, and intraneural metastases.

Symptomatology

When the tumor is localized in the limbs, the first symptom is a slow growing, painless swelling, of hard-elastic consistency, movable in relation to the deep levels.

After the first symptoms, an irritative symptomatology of the affected nerve occurs, characterized by painful paresthesias, burning, tingling, painful crisis, similar to an electric discharge. Such disorders increase by compression or simply by skimming the swelling, or by limb fatigue. Motility disorders are rare and delayed.

The neurological physical signs are tardy and depend on the grade of the tumoral damage present on the nerve. The osteotendinous reflexes are generally decreased, and rarely absent. We can find deficit of sensitivity

Fig. 13.17. Thigh NMR. Sciatic nerve neurinoma

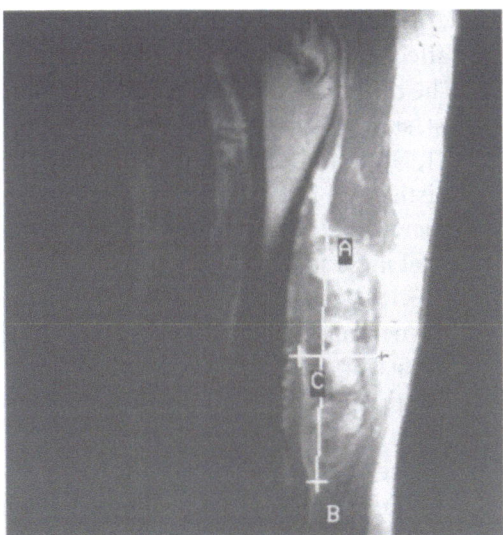

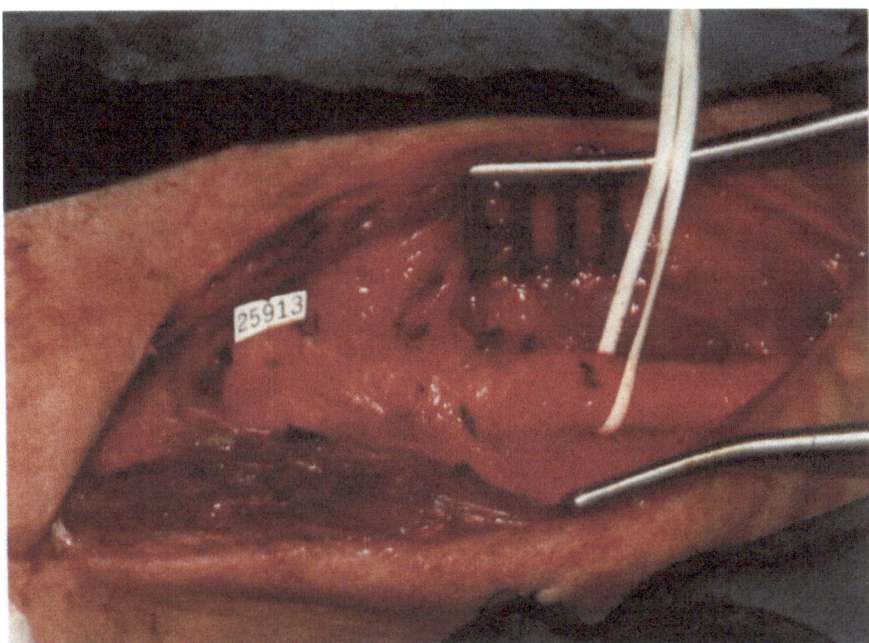

Fig 13.18. Intraoperative aspect of nerve sciatic neuroma

and, rarely, vasomotor disorders in the cutaneous territory innervated by the affected nerve. In most cases, the decrease in strength is slight.

The diagnosis, mainly clinical and completed with an electromyographic test, shows signs of stress and degeneration of the affected nerve.

CT, NMR and echography show the lesions in their morphologic characteristics and in relation to nearby structures (Fig. 13.17).

Theraphy is surgical and consists in the enucleation and removal of the tumoral mass sparing, when possible, the fascicles of the unaffected nerves (Fig. 13.18). When the tumor totally surrounds the nerve, it is necessary to cut the nervous trunk and reconstruct it with termino-terminal anastomosis, in case of a modest gap, or with using the sural nerve grafting.

The prognosis is good for benign tumors, while the malignant tumors relapse in a short time.

In case of *endothoracic localizations*, the diagnosis is mainly accidental, due to the fact that specific signs are often missing. Patients report cough and dyspnea, caused by the mechanical action of the neoplastic mass on the pulmonary parenchyma or on the bronchi.

An important diagnostic element, which appears only in a few cases, is the appearance of painful paresthesias with intercostal irradiation, which increase with deep inspirations, a sign of involvement of the intercostal nerve.

The diagnosis is based on the endothoracic localization and on CT, NMR and echographic studies.

14. Vertebrospinal traumas

In the past, vertebrospinal traumas were rare and were usually due to work and war injuries, or accidental falls. In the last few years, the traumatic spinal pathologies have increased with the concomitant development of motorization.

The incidence is above 30-40 cases a year for one million inhabitants. The most involved age range is 15-24 years, with a decrease in middle age and an increase after 55 years. The incidence, in relation to the causes of the traumatic lesions, can be divided into:
– Traffic accidents (30%-50%)
– Work injuries (20%-40%)
– Sport accidents (7%).

Biomechanics of the vertebral column

The vertebral column (rachis) is formed by an osteo-arthromusculoligamentous structure, and it provides support for the head and the various parts of the trunk. It extends longitudinally from the head, with which it is articulated, as far as the pelvis (Fig. 14.1).

The *osseous component* is formed by the vertebrae. The vertebrae are formed by a body and an arch (or posterior wall). In the arch, there are two peduncles, two articular masses, two laminae and a spinous process.

The *articular apparatus* is formed by the articular body and the articular masses.

The *ligamentous system* is formed by the anterior longitudinal ligament, posterior longitudinal ligament, disk fibrous ring, articular capsulae,

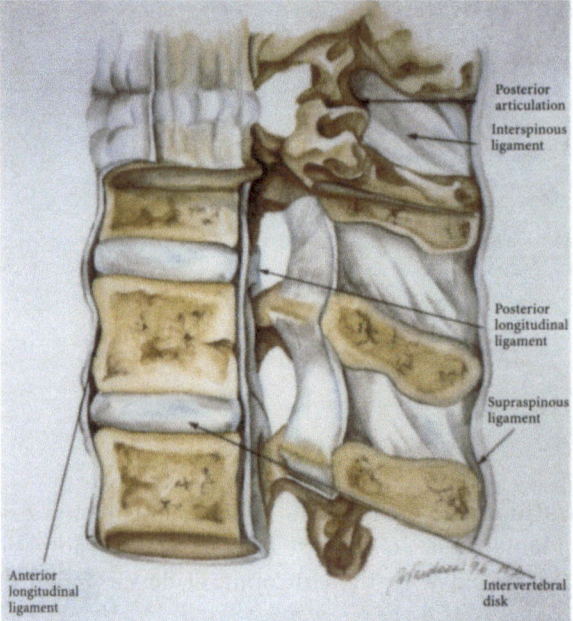

Fig. 14.1. Osteo-artroligamentous structure of the vertebral column

(Figure labels: Posterior articulation; Interspinous ligament; Posterior longitudinal ligament; Supraspinous ligament; Anterior longitudinal ligament; Intervertebral disk)

supraspinous, interspinous and intertransverse ligaments, and yellow ligament.

The *muscular apparatus* is formed by muscles with origin and insertion in the vertebral column. These are the muscles of the vertebral groove or erector muscles of the spine, mainly localized dorsally to the vertebral column, and the intrinsic pre-vertebral and sacrococcygeal muscles localized ventrally.

The standard rachis biomechanics implies that the different articulations must be balanced among them at the same time. Two contiguous vertebrae are maintained in equilibrium, at the level of the intervertebral space and articulations, by the fibroligamentous-capsular and muscular systems. This phenomenon occurs in every mobile segment of the rachis, during standing and movements in the thre-dimensional space. A spinal trauma can cause loss of balance among the normal relationships of the osteoligamentous structures, with consequent vertebral instability. Several authors have attempted to identify the most important anatomical element for the biomechanics of the rachis in order to explain the instability physiopathological mechanisms. A complete neuroradiological examination allows the identification of three types of lesions, potentially responsible for instability:

- Osseous lesions,
- Ligamentous lesions,
- Osteoligamentous lesions.

Denis, in relation to the spinal biomechanical studies by Wute and Panjabi, has divided the rachis into three columns:

- *Anterior column:* anterior longitudinal ligament, fibrous ring anterior part, and vertebral body anterior half.
- *Medial column:* posterior longitudinal ligament, fibrous ring posterior part, and vertebral body posterior half.
- *Posterior column:* posterior osseous arch, posterior ligamentous complex (supra- and interspinous ligament, yellow ligament, articular capsule).

Denis considers the medial column of the utmost importance for the judgement of the fracture instability. The lesion of medial column, if associated with one of the other two columns, causes instability.

Fracture classification

We can distinguish: myelinic and amyelinic fractures, depending on the damage inflicted on the spinal cord by the osseous lesions. The following classification is the most favored, mainly because it is simple and links the type of fracture with its mechanical causes.

- Compression fractures
  - Crush fractures,
  - Burst fractures.
- Pure flexion fractures
  - Anterior fracture or cuneus fracture,
  - Lateral fracture or lateral cuneus fracture.
- Pure extension fractures
  - Tear drop fractures.
- Dislocation fractures
  - Flexion and rotation,
  - Flexion and distortion (seat-belt fractures),
  - Extension and rotation (shear fractures).

Compression fractures

The traumatic force is perpendicular to the vertebral body, which is crushed uniformly with decrease in height. The indirect trauma can be due to a fall from above, without curvature of the spinal vertical axis. Generally, these fractures involve the cervical and lumbar spinal segments. In relation to the trauma intensity, we can classify the compression fractures into crush and burst fractures.

Crush fractures

The traumatic force is perpendicular to the vertebral body, causing uniform decrement in height with compact bone collapsing into the spongious bone below. The fracture is stable because it only causes anterior column alterations (Fig. 14.2). The plain films show, in the lateral projection, decrement in height of the vertebral body and compact bone herniation in the spongious bone.

Burst fractures

The traumatic force is more intense and causes the burst of the vertebral body with comminuted fractures. The fracture is stable if it involves only the anterior column; if the medial column is also affected, with osseous fragments migrating into the spinal canal, the fracture is instable (Fig. 14.3).

The lateral projection of the plain films show decrement in height of the vertebral body and multiple fractures of the vertebral body. In the antero-posterior projection, the plain films can show an increase of the interpeduncular space.

Pure flexion fractures

The traumatic force pushes forward the vertebral column, forming a kyphotic arch. The cervical and dorsolumbar (D12-L1) tracts, the most mobile regions of the vertebral column, receive the greatest traumatic insult. In this instance, the vertebral body is crushed between the above and below metamers, causing an anterior cuneo fracture (Fig. 14.4). A lateral traumatic force causes a lateral cuneo fracture. These are stable fractures because only the anterior column is involved (the posterior column is rarely affected). This type of fracture is due to vertex traumas with the head flexed, car collisions, or dives into shallow water.

The plain films, in lateral projecton, show the compression of the anterior wall of the vertebral body. The cortical flats are usually intact, and there is no considerable increase of the interpeduncular space.

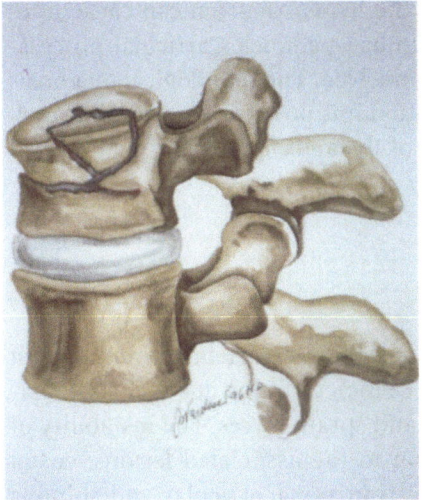
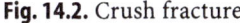

Fig. 14.2. Crush fracture

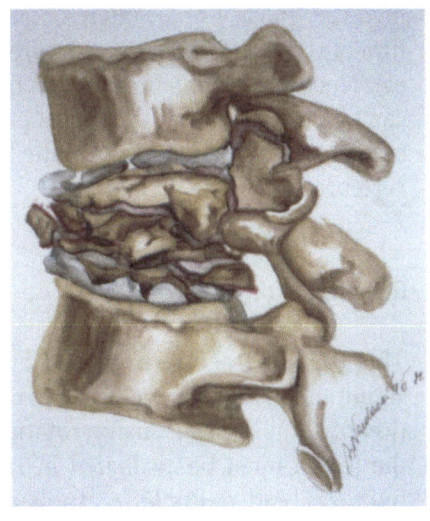

Fig. 14.3. Burst fracture

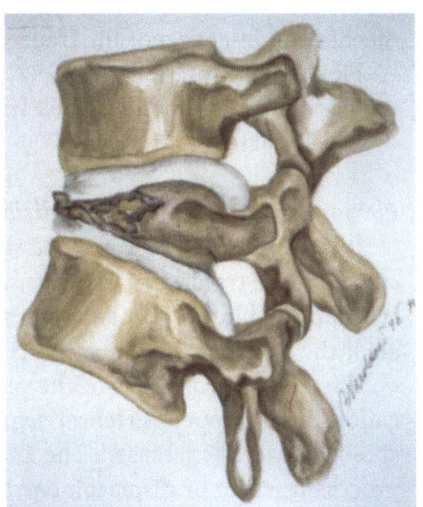

Fig. 14.4. Cuneus fracture

Pure extension fractures

The hyperextension is due to frontal or facial traumas (road collisions, dives into water). The hyperextension causes a forced lordosis with anterior and posterior longitudinal ligament lacerations and wrench fracture of the vertebral body at the level of the upper or lower angle anterior edge ("tear drop fracture"). It is a stable fracture because only the anterior column is involved. In case of an intense trauma, the hyperextension can cause fracture of the posterior arch structures (laminae, peduncles, articular processes). The cervical vertebrae are the most involved. The radiological diagnosis can be difficult, but in the lateral projection it is possible to identify a small osseous fractured fragment at the level of the anterior edge of the involved vertebra.

Dislocation fractures

This type of fracture is caused by a considerable vertebral trauma, with simultaneous involvement of the three Denis's columns due to a combination of compressive, tensive, rotational and sprain forces. The instability of the lesion must be evaluated in relation to the associated lesions: costal fractures, and multiple fractures of the transverse, articular and spinous processes, and of the laminae. The plain films show subluxation and dislocation with vertebral fractures.

We can distinguish three types of fracture-dislocation in relation to the mechanism of action of the trauma:
- Flexion and rotation
- Flexion and sprain (seat-belt fractures)
- Shear fractures.

Flexion and rotation fracture dislocation

It is an instable fracture. The simultaneous flexion and rotation induce considerable transverse displacement. The vertebral body can be cuneus crushed or obliquely broken. The articular processes can break or can luxate if the ligaments are involved (Fig. 14.5).

The lateral projection of the plain films show a subluxation and dislocation of the upper vertebral segment on the vertebra below. The interspinous space is increased. The anteroposterior projections show articular process fracture or displacement, scarce alignment of the peduncles, spinous processes and transverse process fracture.

Flexion and sprain or seat belt fracture-dislocation

This is a fracture due to anterior, medial and posterior column sprains, with the anterior column acting as a hinge (Fig. 14.6). In relation to the trauma intensity, the lesion can involve the osseous component (Chance's fracture) or the ligamentous component, with or without considerable translation. In the first case, there is instability associated with neurological deficits, dural laceration and damage to the endoabdominal organs.

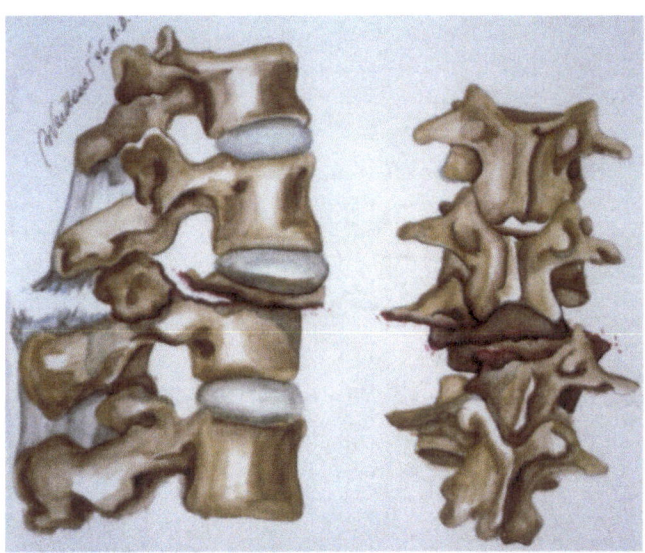

Fig. 14.5. Dislocation fracture due to flexorotation

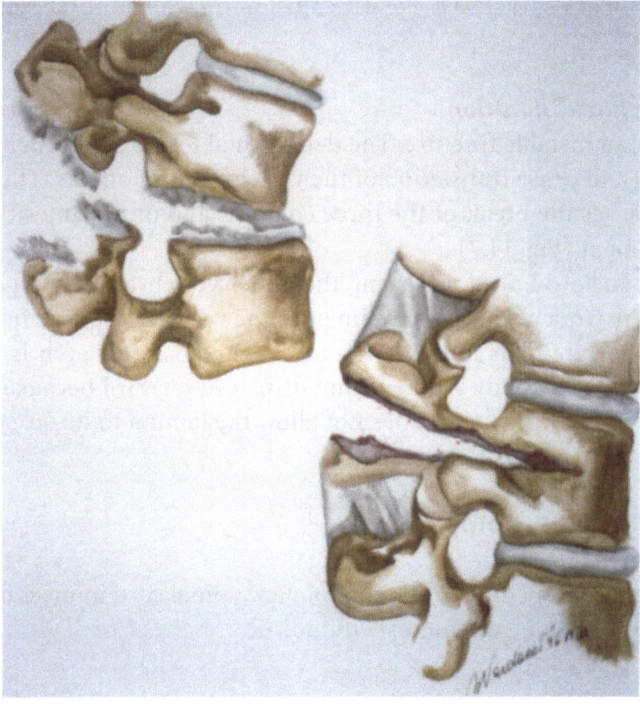

Fig. 14.6. Dislocation fracture (seat-belt fracture) of the osseous and soft tissue (disk and ligamentum)

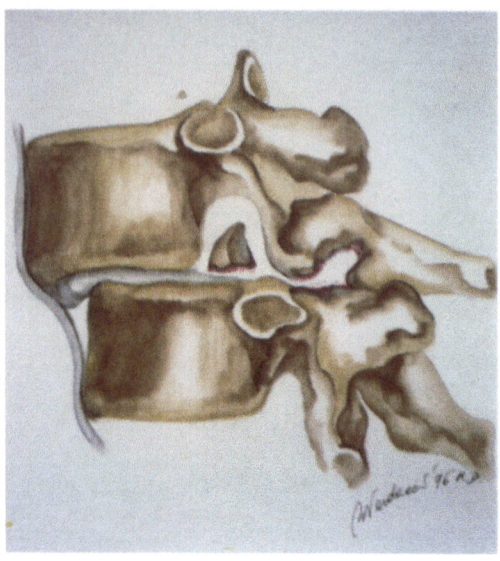

Fig. 14.7. Postero-anterior dislocation-fracture, sheer type

This fracture is characteristic of car collisions in which the passengers wear a seat belt.

Shear fracture dislocation

This is an instable fracture. The detrimental forces are perpendicular to the rachis and cause translation of the vertebral components. The traumatic force causes the break of the three columns and of the anterior longitudinal ligament (Fig. 14.7).

In the postero-anterior variant, the upper vertebral body segments are displaced in front of the lower segments. The vertebral body is intact, while the posterior arch has multiple fractures. The posterior arch is separated from the vertebral body segment, and displaced forward because the vertical orientation of the facets does not allow the lamina to do so.

Pathological anatomy

From an anatomopathological point of view, spinal cord injuries due to vertebral trauma can be distinguished into:
- Spinal concussion
- Spinal contusion
- Spinal laceration
- Hematomyelia.

Spinal concussion

It is due to a temporary spinal functional injury. Usually, there are no anatomical lesions, but in some cases necrosis and hemorrhagic foci can be found with a moderate interstitial edema and nerve fibers demyelination. Clinically, there is a complete but temporary interruption of the spinal functions below the lesion level.

Spinal contusion

It is due to a short compression on the spinal cord. Macroscopically, the spinal cord appears normal or pale, increased in volume by two or three times. In the white and gray matter, there are necrosis and hemorrhagic foci with considerable edema, and ascending and descending nervous tract demyelination.

Spinal laceration

It is a spinal lesion due to considerable trauma, causing vertebral body luxation, sliding and fracture. The dura and arachnoid are lacerated. The spinal cord is totally interrupted or altered by necrotic-hemorrhagic foci and considerable edema. These foci evolve into meningospinal scars, due to neuroglia and connective tissue proliferation.

Hematomyelia

It is a blood collection due to the breakage arterial and venous vessels. It can be localized at the level of the contusive focus or at a distance. The cervical spine is more often involved.

Symptomatology

The vertebrospinal trauma symptomatology depends both on skeletal lesions and neurological complications. Skeletal lesion symptomatology is characterized by:
- Spontaneous or induced pain at the level of the fracture focus
- Rachis stiffness

- Antalgic muscular contracture
- Rachis acute angle deformity or gibbus
- Slight fever for few days.

Clinically, post-traumatic spinal lesions, in relation to their size, can be distinguished into:
- Complete section syndrome
- Incomplete section syndrome
- Radicular section syndrome.

Complete section syndrome

It is due to spinal concussion or contusion or less often to spinal compression or section. During the initial phase, there are no elements to determine if the non-functionality of the spinal cord is due to an anatomical interruption or to a temporary functional interruption (spinal shock). The clinical syndrome is variable and depends on the evolution and the time when the patient is examined. The complete section syndrome can be distinguished into three phases:
a) Initial (or spinal shock) phase
b) Spinal shock recovery or resolution phase
c) Stabilization phase

Initial (or spinal shock) phase

MOTOR DISORDERS
- Flaccid paraplegia or tetraplegia in relation to cervical or dorsolumbar lesions. The patient is in bed, with the upper limbs pronated and lower limbs extended and slightly extrarotated.
- Muscular atony.
- Deep reflex abolition.
- Skin reflex abolition.
- The anal and cremasteric reflexes can be preserved due to a precocious automatic activity of the medullary cone.

SENSORIAL DISORDERS
- Total anesthesia below the lesion, with involvement of all sensory modalities (thermal, painful, tactile, position sense, pallesthesia).

VEGETATIVE DISORDERS
- Vasomotor disorders: a cutaneous vasomotor reaction appears, characterized by face and neck blush, head and shoulder profuse sweating, and

serious and sometimes drug resistant arterial hypotension. The higher the spinal lesion, the more serious the disorder is.

- Thermic regulation disorders: there is considerable thermic instability. Usually, the temperature increases in the regions below the lesion. The temperature can reach 38°-38,5° C. This hyperthermia is not easily controlled with medications.
- Vescical disorders: vescical retention and distension.
- Rectal disorders: fecal retention due to the intestinal atony, and sometimes incontinence.
- Cutaneous trophism disorders: cutaneous ulcerations occur precociously.
- Precocious abdominal syndrome: this syndrome, described for the first time in 1920 by Guillain-Barré, is characterized by meteorism, vomiting, and hiccup due to a paralytic ileus.
- Pulmonary complications: dyspnea, cyanosis due to bronchial hypersecretion, pulmonary congestion, and pulmonary edema. These complications mainly affect patients with dorsal trauma (D1-D7).

Spinal shock recovery or resolution phase

The spinal shock phase persists from three days to three weeks. When the shock disappears, the spinal functions resume and the degree of recovery is related to the spinal cord anatomical damage caused by the trauma. In relation to the severity of the spinal lesion, we can distinguish two syndromes: complete section spinal syndrome and incomplete section spinal syndrome.

Complete section spinal syndrome

Paraplegia and total anesthesia remain stationary.

The abdominal and cremasteric reflexes reappear, together with the cutaneous defense reflex of the flexor muscles of the lower limbs (defense or triple flexion reflex).

The automatic reflex activity reappears. We can observe automatic movements, simulating spontaneous movements. The bladder and rectum can recover an automatic activity.

The genital activity is modified: there is no spontaneous erection or priapism, but the erection can be obtained stimulating the glans and nearby mucosa. Ejaculation is possible, but the sperm are rarely fertile. Ulcers must be closely monitored because they can become deeper, especially at the level of the sacrum and heel.

Incomplete section syndrome

In relation to the size and topography of the spinal injury caused by verte-
brospinal trauma, we can distinguish several incomplete spinal syndromes:
- Spinal hemisection syndrome or Brown-Séquard's syndrome,
- Posterior transverse hemisection or Roussy and Lhermitte's syndrome,
- Anterior spinal suffering syndrome or Schneider's syndrome,
- Centro-spinal suffering syndrome or Schneider's syndrome.

Brown-Séquard's syndrome
It is due to the complete interruption of the right or left half of the
spinal cord. From a clinical point of view, this is a dissociated syndrome
characterized by the following disorders ipsilateral to the lesion:
- Voluntary motility paralysis caused by pyramidal tract interruption.
- Deep sensory loss (posture sense, vibratory, discriminating tactile, and
  spatial sensitivity, tactile localization) due to the posterior cord interruption.
- Vasodilation due to half body vasoparalysis.

Contralateral to the lesion, there is motility and deep sensory preservation while there is tactile, thermal and painful anesthesia below the lesion,
due to corticospinal tract interruption. In the metamer innervated by the
injured spinal segments, there is severe general hypoesthesia and hyperes-
thesia in the metamer above.

Posterior transverse hemisection syndrome or roussy-lhermitte's syndrome
It is due to posterior cords, posterior horns and posterior part of the lat-
eral cords elective section. Clinically, this syndrome is characterized by:
- Paraplegia or paraparesis with reflex abolition,
- Abolition or serious involvement of deep sensory functions,
- More or less complete superficial sensory preservation,
- Dejerine's radicular fiber syndrome.

Schneider's anterior spinal suffering syndrome
It is an acute syndrome clinically characterized by:
- Severe paraplegia or paraparesis below the lesion
- Hypoalgesia with frequent preservation of the tactile and vibratory sen-
  sitivities.

Centro-spinal suffering syndrome or schneider's syndrome
This syndrome involves the cervical spine. It is due to an anterior spinal

compression, causing microscopic and punctiform hemorrhagic lesions and, sometimes, gray matter hematomyelia. This syndrome can be due to circulatory alterations in the regions of the anterior spinal artery. Clinically, this syndrome is characterized by:
- Motor deficits of the limbs, mainly upper limbs,
- Sensory disorders, mainly of the thermal and painful sensitivities,
- Sphincteric disorders (retention).
  This syndrome improves during the days following the trauma.

Radicular lesion syndrome

This is a nerve root lesion occuring in both the intraforaminal tract and the exit zone from the spinal cord (avulsion). The most involved areas are the cervical and lumbar regions.

Radiology of vertebral fractures

The radiological evaluation of vertebral fractures has been modified by the introduction of CT, NMR, and hydrosoluble contrast medium. The plain films are still an important screening examination of trauma because they show vertebral fractures and probable dislocation (Fig. 14.8).

CT achieves a best visualization of the posterior vertebral arch, articular facets, body and spinal canal, and allows the reconstruction of the coronal, sagittal, axial and oblique planes. CT implies less risks for the patient in comparison to conventional multiplanar stratigraphy that requires constant mobility (Fig. 14.9).

Myelography with metrizamide, utilized in patients with neurological deficit not corresponding to the level or size of the vertebral injury, has been completely replaced by NMR. Spinal NMR shows spinal injuries (contusion, laceration, hematoma, edema) and allows a more precise definition of the prognosis (Fig. 14.10).

Vertebrospinal lesion therapy

The treatment of patients affected by vertebrospinal trauma varies in relation to the different evolutive phases (Table 14.1). The initial aim is to preserve the patient's life, with prompt treatment of shock, precocious respiratory disorders, acute abdominal syndrome, urinary retention and ther-

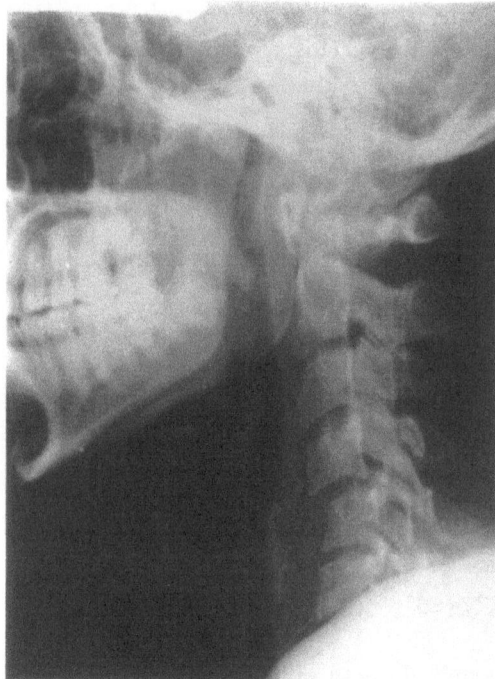

Fig. 14.8. Post-traumatic spondylolisthesis of C4 on C5. Cervical X-ray, lateral view

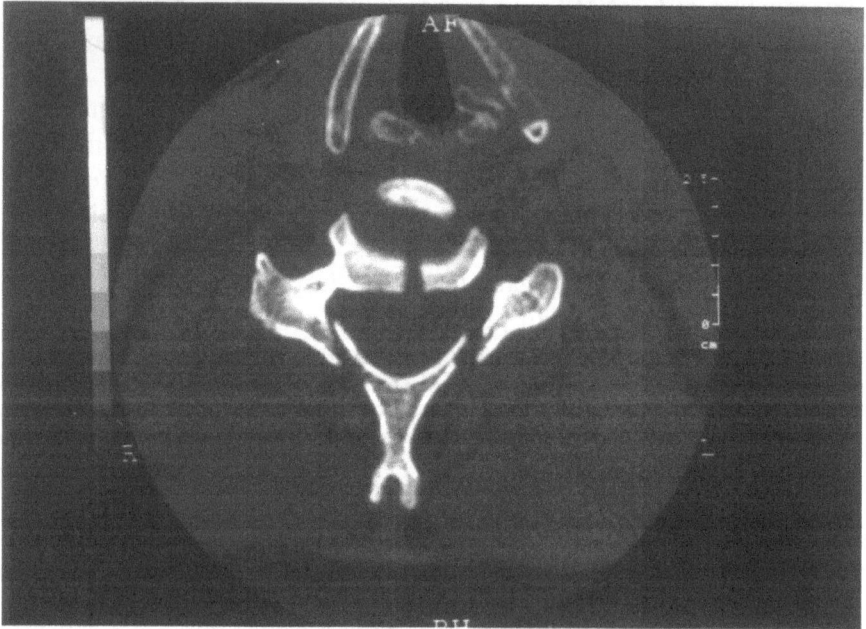

Fig. 14.9. Multiple cervical fractures. Cervical CT (bone window). Multiple lines of
fracture at vertebral body and laminae level

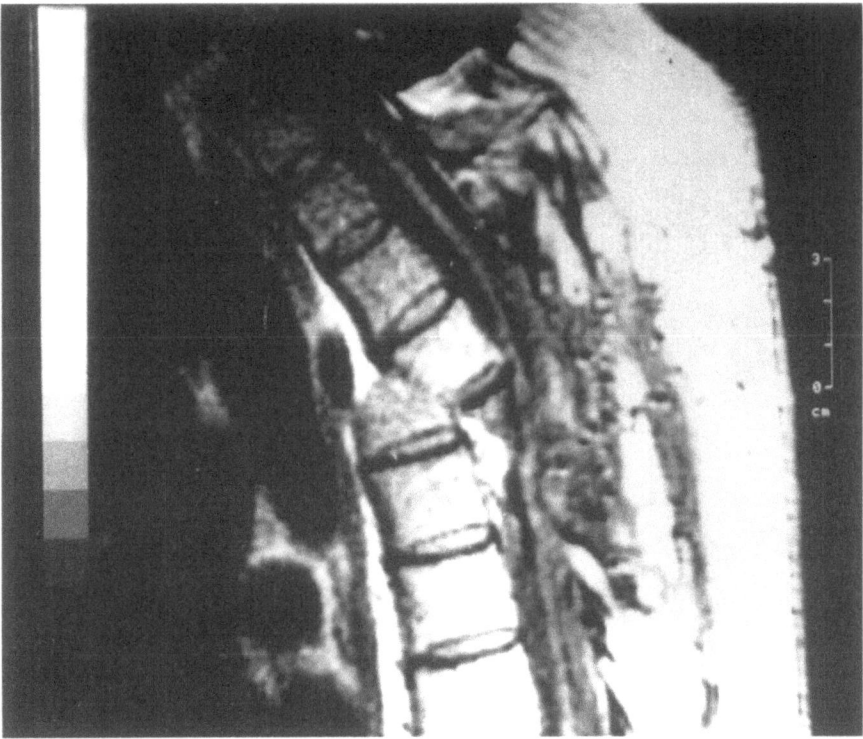

Fig. 14.10. Vertebrodorsal fracture. MRI, T1-weighted images, sagittal view. Decomposed vertebral fracture with posterior displacement of the vertebral body superior part and spinal cord compression

Table 14.1. Aims of therapy for vertebrospinal trauma

– Prevent pulmonary, gastrointestinal and genitourinary complications
– Preserve the residual medullar functions
– Achieve neurological recovery
– Realign the vertebral column
– Stabilize the vertebral column
– Early rehabilitation

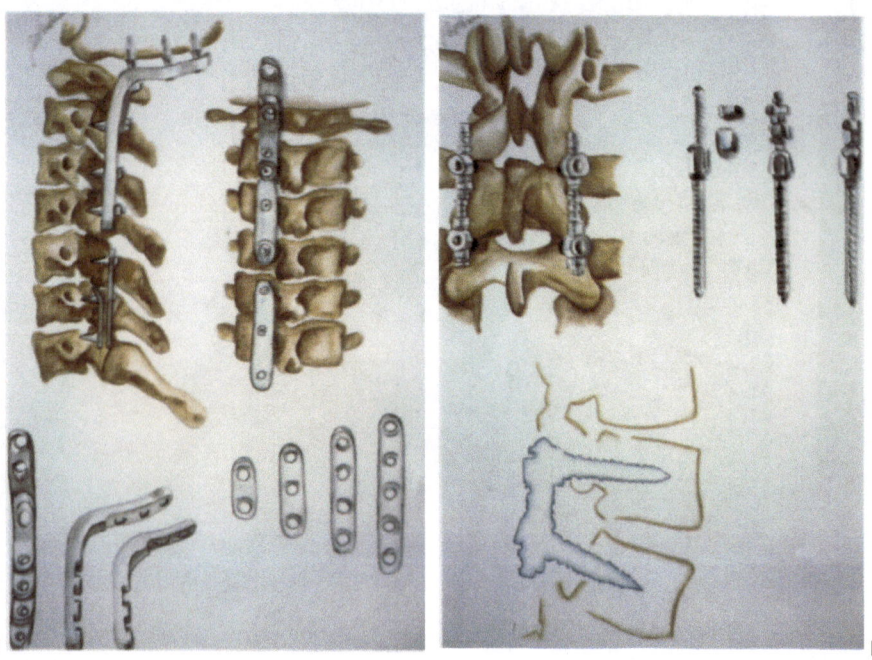

a   b

Fig. 14.11. a Transpedicular posterior fixation system. **b** Transpeduncular posterior fixation system

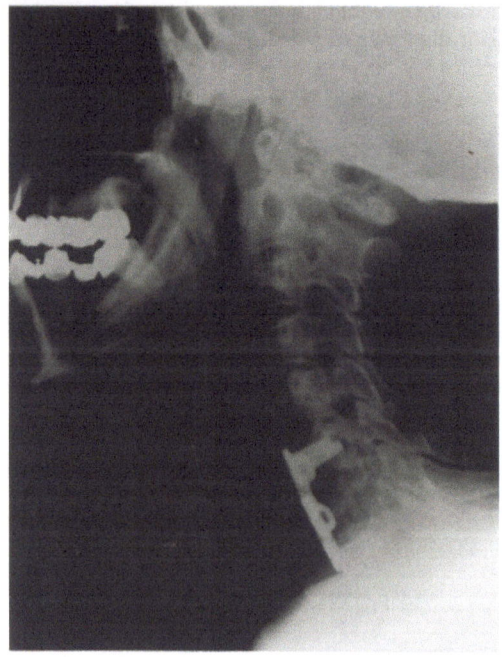

Fig. 14.12. Cervical X-ray. Anterior fixation of a C6-C7 instable fracture

mocoagulation disorders. Subsequently, it is necessary to preserve the neurological functions with an appropriate and precocious vertebral column decompression and stabilization. This treatment can be conservative or surgical.

Conservative therapy

Rest and support from corsets and neck collars are sufficent if the fracture is stable and there are no spinal or radicular lesions.

Surgical therapy

If the fracture is unstable, with or without spinal lesions, it is necessary to decompress the spinal cord and the roots compressed by osseous fragments, diskal fragments, or hematomas. A posterior approach (laminectomy) or anterolateral approach to remove the nervous structure compression can be employed, in order to reduce and realign the fractured vertebrae with a traction or surgical reduction. Finally, the fractured vertebrae are stabilized with metal plates, bars (Fig. 14.11-14.13) wires and osseous grafts.

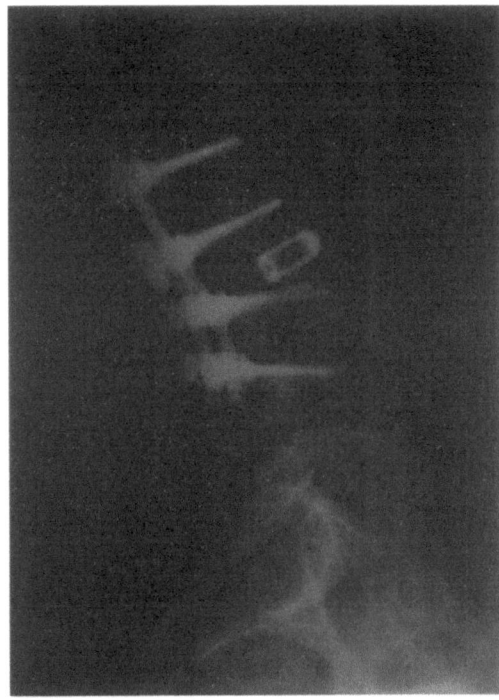

Fig. 14.13. Lumbosacral X-ray, lateral view, of a patient treated for post-traumatic spondylolisthesis. Presence of metallic plates and screws in vertebral bodies. Titanium cage at L2-L3 level

Treatment of sequelae

If, despite spinal and nervous root decompression and vertebrae realignment and fixation, the neurological deficits persist, an equipe of specialists is necessary (neurosurgeons, orthopedics, urologists, plastic surgeons, and physiotherapists) to allow:

- Motor rehabilitation
- Treatment of urinary complications
- Ulcer treatment
- Contracture treatment
- Pain treatment